GENTLE GIANTS

GENTLE GIANTS

*The powerful story of one woman's
unconventional struggle against breast cancer*

PENNY BROHN

CENTURY PUBLISHING

LONDON

Copyright © Penny Brohn 1986

First published in Great Britain in 1986
by Century Hutchinson Limited
Brookmount House, 62–65 Chandos Place,
Covent Garden, London WC2N 4NW

British Library Cataloguing in Publication Data

Brohn, Penny
    Gentle giants: the powerful story of one
    woman's unconventional struggle against cancer.
    1. Cancer—Treatment
    I. Title
    616.99'406   RC270.8

ISBN 0 7126 1132 0

Printed in Great Britain in 1985 by
St Edmundsbury Press, Bury St Edmunds, Suffolk
Bound by Butler & Tanner Ltd, Frome, Somerset

Contents

Dedication

My childhood was full of giants. My father's speciality was a wonderful line in bedtime stories that featured a couple of giants whose sole purpose in life seemed to be rescuing myself and my sisters from the various dangers and perils of our daring exploits. My giants were always kind and brave. We didn't go in for the Fee-Fi-Fo-Fum variety.

This book is dedicated to the men and women who were kind enough and brave enough to come to my aid later in my life, when the myth became reality:
Dr. Josef Issels
Dr. Alec Forbes
Dr. Ainslie Meares
The Rev Tim Tiley
Dr. Dorothy West
Dr. Ernesto Contreras
Dr. Hans Moolenberg
Dr. Norman Howard
And of course David (who might have wished for an easier life) grew to be the kindest AND gentlest of them all. Thanks and thanks and ever thanks.

Introduction

This is a book about a process, not an event: a healing not a cure. It is about the business of growing up. Because this process didn't really start in me until I got cancer then, inevitably, the subject of cancer looms large throughout the book, but it is significant only in so far as it precipitated a dramatic re-shuffling of my life and a rapid rate of change. You don't have to have cancer for this to happen to you, any crisis will do.

I have tried to write about the peripheral effects of having cancer because these are the shared aspects of any life crisis, and I have tried to avoid too much detail about the illness itself. It's the dis-ease that is interesting, not the disease.

When things are going well for us we are usually able to deny or thrust away from ourselves the dark and dreadful side of our existence. In our early childhood we shape a life-plan for ourselves that does not include fear and pain, despair and helplessness. Often, when something so dreadful happens that we finally get swept up in such things, we find we have few, if any, mechanisms for coping with them. For some of my friends their crisis was the death of a baby, for another the loss of a limb. For me it was having cancer. For nearly all of us there comes a moment when we are overwhelmed by the negative side of life, and by and large, we don't know how to handle it. I felt hopelessly inadequate and ill-equipped for the task of dealing with a life-threatening disease and was constantly looking for help. I have dedicated this book to the people who were big enough and strong enough to help me.

They needed to be big and strong because, since my crisis was manifesting itself as a physical disease, I was looking for help mainly amongst doctors and physical therapists.

Anyone operating in this field has spent years of their lives studying one particular way of treating illness: it may be holistic, allopathic, homeoepathic, conventional, alternative, young or old, but it is a system and it has a method. By the time a practitioner gets to qualify in any one of these systems he has invested a lot of himself in the process of learning it and naturally the model of medicine that he has acquired becomes very precious to him. He is not going to question it lightly.

I realise, with all the wisdom of hindsight, that when I came flying out of the woodwork, full of ideas about cancerous personalities, cancerous relationships, and existential crises, I appeared as a challenge and a threat to any medical model that saw cancer only as a cellular aberration. It was my good fortune to be able to find men and women who were tough enough and far-sighted enough to be flexible about their model of disease. Some of them had broken out of the mould years before I met them and were already ploughing a vigorous and expansive furrow through fresh fields. Joseph Issels and Hans Moolenberg for example. But for others this was a new way of dealing with a cancer patient and it must have been hard. This was outside their usual model, something not taught at medical school. Like me, they were learning as they went.

That's always the snag of course: you have to make it up as you go along. No time for practising or extra rehearsals. This is it. It's happening now. Cancer or no cancer, this life is the real thing.

Chapter 1

The whole earth is our hospital
Endowed by the ruined millionaire,
Wherein, if we do well, we shall
Die of the absolute paternal care
That will not leave us, but prevents us everywhere.
                                                    T.S. Eliot

The only remarkable thing about the flight to Germany was the fact that I wasn't frightened. Not frightened, that is, of looking out of the plane and seeing the wings actually flapping through the turbulence. My small grasp of aerodynamics suggested to me that whereas birds' wings need to flap most of the time, aeroplane wings are designed to do so only in emergencies. Judging by the facial contortions of my fellow passengers and the honey-smooth reassurances of the air-hostess, this might well have been an emergency, but I wasn't frightened. There was a very simple reason for this: I had used up my fear quotient. I had been so frightened for the previous week or two I had exhausted my capacity to react fearfully to anything except the fact that I had cancer.

I was frightened all right, but not of crash-landing into the sea.

How do you feel when someone tells you you have cancer? I've been asked this question so many times it must be an area of considerable interest to a lot of people. I have some difficulty in answering it because the first thought that overwhelmed me at the time was that – regardless of whatever emotional response was welling up inside me – I must not let my feelings show. In true British style I braced myself, recalled years of authoritarian admonitions not to 'carry on' or 'make a fuss' and replied mildly with something like, 'Oh dear, I thought it might be.'

Eavesdropping later on a conversation between my informant and the ward sister I heard that I had 'taken it very well'. I had not in fact taken it at all well, although from his point of view it had all gone quite smoothly. I hadn't raged and cried and given him a hard time, or adopted the historical Greek style of murdering him on the spot just for being the bearer of such grim tidings, so from his point of view things had gone quite well. His management of my crisis consisted of a pat on the hand and the assurance that he was very sorry. I was glad he was very sorry. I was pretty sorry myself. I imagined everyone would be sorry – it seemed inconceivable to me that any reasonable human being wouldn't be very sorry. I didn't think very sorry was worth much. That left me with a pat on the hand. Not enough. Not nearly enough.

Would it have been any different if I had screamed and torn at the sheets? I think not. At least, not in terms of human contact and counselling, although there were tranquillisers at the ready in the event of just such a performance.

It was all oddly reminiscent of when my parents had died: if you cried someone told you to pull yourself together, if you kept calm someone said you ought to have a good cry. The only certainty was that nobody knew quite what to do, merely responding with a sort of jittery caution, as if death were such a rare and unexpected event one would never anticipate getting tangled up in it oneself or having to cope with someone who was. The person who told me I had cancer did so as if he had never done such a thing before and would not expect to do so again. Although the former might have been true, the latter almost certainly was not. It was a depressingly inadequate encounter.

So, it's hard to say accurately what I felt. I only know that the feelings were massive and overwhelming, and that when I talk now to people who describe how frightened they were I can identify with that, but I can identify too with the person who admits to anger, panic, even guilt. I felt all of these things.

2

For me, and for many others, being told you have cancer evokes a crisis, an event of an altogether different magnitude from that experienced by one's fellow-patients waiting to recover from the shock and trauma of their hospital experiences. The crisis for the cancer patient is the knowledge that he may never recover.

This is the ultimate existential crisis and it packs a terrific punch. The problem of coping with it, for me, came partly from the fact that nobody else was acknowledging the magnitude of my shock. My medical team were dealing with the diagnosis as a physical problem in terms of their personal and technological resources, while I was trying to handle it on a mental and emotional level as a spiritual challenge. This fundamental difference between the hospital's view of the situation and my own widened as the days went by. Every white-coated visitor to my bedside came bearing details of surgical techniques, advances in radiotherapy and so on, while I burbled on about stress and why I thought I was ill.

It seemed incredible to me that whatever attention had previously been afforded to me generally was now withdrawn and focused exclusively on my left breast. Doctors, studiously avoiding eye contact, came, examined me, and left.

Communications started breaking down on all fronts. My nervous attempts to discuss holistic treatment resulted only in the doctors becoming more aggressive in the promotion of their own proposals and, sadly, just a little threatening. This was all the more disappointing in view of that fact that my idea of holistic treatment at that time was to have someone refer to me by name – and not as 'a grade one carcinoma of the left breast', which had happened more than once – also to listen to some of the chaos that was churning through my mind.

Meanwhile my relationship with the rest of the ward changed too. Women who had stopped to talk before the deadly diagnosis was made, subsequently tip-toed past the end of my bed, eyes fixed full ahead. Any fears they may have had for their own safety were now, in a sense, being borne by

3

me. The statistical quota had been filled, the scapegoat selected. Scapegoats are, by definition, pushed out of the fold.

How did I feel? I felt lonely, frightened and outcast, but I also felt a new kind of awareness. Slowly, in the midst of all the chaos and background noise, my intuition and perception deepened and I found myself looking at and listening to my doctors, my family and my friends with a slight degree of detachment, knowing that they were not party to this and sensing that I must temper their responses to the new, sharper edge of my understanding.

The most significant feeling I had was that my cancer involved the whole of me, not just a bumpy bit on the left-hand side going down. Something had gone fundamentally wrong with me, I knew I was off course, and that whatever treatment I had would need to involve some redirecting if it was to stay effective for long. This was no crazy, cosmic accident, or merely a bit of nonsense from some un-controllable, immature cells. I knew that my cancer was an accumulation of undischarged grief, pent-up guilt and layer upon layer of fear. Somehow having it cut out didn't seem like the ultimate long-term solution. That might get rid of the lump, but would it get rid of the grief, guilt and fear, and if not, then where would they go? Underground for a while I had no doubt, only to re-emerge later as another lump somewhere else. Wasn't that what happened more often than not to cancer patients? Treated, discharged, declared 'clear', told to go home and forget all about it, only to reappear with secondaries in a few years' time.

Naturally I had considerable difficulty in expressing this to any of the doctors – who were now arriving in pairs, then in groups and finally in whole teams, in the effort to talk some sense into this awkward patient. It didn't help that hours of silent weeping had left me thick-headed and inarticulate, barely capable of stringing three or four words together without shedding a few more tears.

I was also handicapped by the fact that my certainty that my cancer was a disease of the whole of me was not matched by any certainty that a violent physical assault on the tumour might not be a good thing. Maybe there was a case for

4

accepting the hospital's offer of an all-out attack in the short term, leaving me free to deal with all the psychological and emotional mess afterwards.

There is no doubt that had anyone at the time shown the smallest degree of understanding, or even interest, in my view of the situation and offered to help, then I would cheerfully have adopted the role that was expected of me, been a model patient and agreed to everything that was suggested. My problem was that I didn't trust myself to get out of my inner turmoil alone and without help.

I strongly suspected that being wheeled off for a mastectomy and facing up to radiotherapy would use all my strength and exhaust my courage. How would I then be able to face the task of grappling with my shadow, facing up to the dark forces that had already overwhelmed me in disease? What reason had I to think that I would suddenly find a way through this painful maze just because I was facing a few hours of traumatic surgery? It was a risk that I did not dare to take. Forming faintly in my mind was the understanding that I needed healing, and that this might not be the same thing as treatment, or even cure.

I was also handicapped by the fact that, not only did my response to having cancer conflict with that of my medical team, but it appeared also to conflict with that of millions of other cancer patients who had accepted their lot with stoic courage, bravely undergone whatever treatment was on offer, and had generally been co-operative. I never for one moment imagined that my response was unique, although it was obvious that other patients who might have felt like me had kept it to themselves. I don't blame them: the role I was playing was painfully difficult. There were many midnight hours when I contemplated peaceful submission to the operating table just to win back the approval, encouragement and sympathy that I longed for, but something always held me back.

In a final, desperate bid for understanding I decided that all this psycho-social drama that nobody had really grasped would have to be clarified. Risking the agony of deep exposure I asked to see the doctor who seemed to have played the role of chief negotiator. He arrived, briskly pleased,

5

imagining no doubt that I had finally come to see things his way.

'I think I know why I'm ill,' I announced.

It seems funny now that I should have expected this to elicit any response other than the one I got, but I was absolutely shattered by his exasperated reply.

'Well, that doesn't make any difference to the way we treat you.'

I understand much better now how tightly some people are welded to a mechanistic model of disease which makes such attitudes entirely predictable, but having spent a good part of my life trying to disentangle myself from this narrow, linear view of medicine by the simple expedient of training as an acupuncturist, I knew I had to find medical help from someone whose ideas matched up a little more closely with my own.

I also knew that the decision I was about to make might prove to be among the most important I should ever make. I needed time to think things through. However, my refusal to accept the proferred mastectomy so infuriated the doctor that he terminated our discussion by sweeping away through the curtains that surrounded my bed, firing as his parting shot over his shoulder: 'The decision will obviously have to be taken out of your hands.'

Not this decision, comrade; not these hands.

Thus it was that I discharged myself from hospital with a huge, weeping haematoma, a big bundle of sterile dressings and not the faintest idea of what I would do next.

One of the first of a stream of visitors to the house was my general medical practitioner. He came incredulous with irritation. What did I think I was doing leaving the hospital? Didn't I know about the wonderful advances in chemo-therapy? (Nobody had mentioned chemotherapy to me until this point and it was not a smart move on his part to raise it then. It served to strengthen my resolve to stay away from hospital a while longer.)

His next contribution to the confusion was to reassure my husband, David, that it was quite safe to continue having sexual relationships with me but, please, to stop encourag-ing me in my rejection of what the hospital had to offer

6

because by so doing, 'You're throwing her life away.

Neither of these offerings was particularly helpful. The first because it had not occurred to either of us that cancer was a contact disease, and the second because David had the greatest of difficulty in keeping up with my ever-changing decisions, never mind finding the strength to support me in any of them. I hopped restlessly from one idea to another; sifting, examining and rejecting, but never staying with anything for long.

I knew, because I had read books about them, that there were people who claimed to have cured their cancers with diet, or massive doses of vitamin C or some sort of mind-over-matter routine. And, to be fair, I knew that there were plenty of people alive and well attributing their survival to the wonders of modern science. But I also knew that none of these techniques was effective in all cases. Make no mistake about it, my stubborn determination to have an existential crisis as well as a lump in my breast was prompted in large part by the fact that nobody had offered me a cure. I think if the hospital had been dealing a good line in lifetime guarantees along with their wares then I would have been just another grateful customer.

Unfortunately I was only too well aware of the prognosis for a middle-aged woman with breast cancer: somewhere around an eighty per cent chance of surviving five years. It didn't seem too bad at first and, during one of the periods when I had decided to take the high technology route, I asked one of the doctors what I could do to help myself. To put myself in the winning half of the statistic.

'Nothing,' he replied.

Within me roared a helpless, desperate king: 'Nothing will come of nothing – speak again!'

But I was speechless and this man had nothing else to add. We sat gazing wordlessly at each other across the abyss, knowing neither of us had the strength to bridge it. Like old Lear and his daughter we were both of us too proud or too frightened to find a more peaceful solution to the impasse, and thus we silently initiated the inexorable unfolding of a much more dramatic scenario.

'Nothing!'

7

How could I take that seriously? There is not one single area of human endeavour that is not influenced by effort. Was the man mad? No madder than I was to walk away from the only source of help that I knew.

More visitors came. With my background in alternative medicine I had high hopes of some really good ideas, but one after another my colleagues backed off into safety: 'I should go along with them if I were you.'

One wonderful night we forgot it all. Loving friends brought champagne which we drank together on our huge brass bed, playing a few rather drunken rubbers of bridge. My first real understanding that it was possible to live in, and enjoy, the present, without bemoaning the past or dreading the future.

And then it came, the first breakthrough: 'What about that man who didn't save Lillian Board?'

Poor, dear Josef Issels. Condemned by the British public to be remembered always for one of his failures, he was constantly referred to me in this way. David rang Directory Enquiries:

'Where does he live?'

'Somewhere in Germany.'

'I'll call you back.'

As indeed they did, with the number ringing out at the other end and, unbelievably, someone who could speak English saying, 'ring tomorrow and you can talk to him.'

'Bring her,' he said. 'Bring her as quickly as possible.'

We found out what we could, which wasn't much. Apparently he treated the whole body, not just the tumour. It sounded hopeful and we decided to go and see.

My doctor returned, irritation giving way to anger. He knew different things about Issels. He paced the bedroom, trying not to shout.

'He's a crook and a charlatan!'

He seemed pretty sure about that, but I had decided to go and see for myself. We bought cheap return tickets, valid for four days, and set off.

The plane finally landed at Munich, the flapping wings having done a very good job, but having cancer seemed a high price to pay for a bit of cool flying sophistication.

8

Future visitors who came to see me in Germany swept away from the airport in Mercedes-chauffeured luxury. Not for them the doubtful, ethnic delights of buses and coaches and the glittering efficiency of Munich railway station. But David had it all worked out: it was actually possible to get to Bad Weissee this way before dark, and of course it would be cheaper. As it turned out only marginally cheaper, but the habits of a lifetime die hard. It was public transport for us.

Waiting for David to check a connection at the railway station I wondered if I might not actually die before we arrived. My breast was sore and painful, I was exhausted by the tension and strain of the previous weeks – perhaps also a little unnerved by the flapping aeroplane wings, who knows. I only know that, standing there, guarding our trolley and few bits of luggage I was suddenly emptied of all strength and overcome with pain and weakness. Afraid that I might actually faint, I lay down on the trolley and rested my head against my suitcase.

This rather bizarre behaviour did not have the same effect in Munich as it might have had at Bath Spa, our point of departure. There I think my fellow-countrymen would have suffered agonies of embarrassment and been forced to use all the avoidance techniques typical of the British to pretend this wasn't happening. No so my Teutonic hosts. Someone tapped me on the shoulder and asked me something, stamping off impatiently when I clearly did not understand. Perhaps he wanted the trolley and felt I was not using it for its proper purpose? Someone else wheeled me a few yards to one side; no doubt because I was blocking the thoroughfare and generally getting in the way. There was definitely a comical side to all this, but I was sinking into a humourless despair. I was afraid and I felt very ill.

I hadn't felt ill like this before. Was I feeling ill because I was afraid, or was I frightened because I was feeling ill?

David rescued me, wheeled me to the train, loaded me on and assured me for the thousandth time that everything would be all right.

I had no choice but to change the dressing on my breast in the lavatory. German trains are moderately clean, but are not designed for this particular use and it was a nerve-wracking procedure. A far cry from the secure, aseptic, sweet-smelling dressing-room at the hospital and I promptly wished I was back there. What was I doing taking such terrible risks? I should look pretty stupid if I died of septicaemia. I could hardly bear to look at my breast it was such a pathetic mess. What a farce that operation had been!

My tumour presented itself in the lower left quadrant of my left breast, although, to talk about 'quadrants' in relation to my breasts is a bit misleading. Apparently breast cancer is more prevalent in women with small breasts, a phenomenon which I do not find in the least bit puzzling because it must be more difficult to find the lumps in big ones.

My first presentation of this two-centimetre-long trouble-maker was to my general practitioner.

'I'm sure it's nothing, but just to be on the safe side I'd like you to see a surgeon.'

My encounter with the surgeon was almost identical.

'I don't think there's anything to worry about here, but just to be sure we'll have it out.'

I argued as best I could. If nobody was very worried, couldn't we leave it for a while? I could come back to the hospital and have it monitored.

'No.'

'But I'm worried about having a general anaesthetic; I've been so run-down lately.'

I so desperately wanted him to take me up on this. There had been quite a few indicators here and there that fed the creeping anxiety that all was not well with me, but I could not have raised these things without encouragement. Outwardly I was trying to convince myself there was nothing wrong; inwardly I felt the need to talk about it and get some helpful advice.

'Don't have a general then, have a local.'

'Good. Right. Lovely, I'll have a local. Can I do it myself with acupuncture?' I admit that was a bit provocative. Provocative, but irrisistible.

'No, you can't!'

As things turned out I couldn't have made a worse mess of it than they did.

I was to be a 'quickie', a five-minute addition at the beginning of the afternoon theatre list. Not even a lumpectomy, but a lump biopsy; in and out in a moment.

Not so.

My lump didn't want to part company with me and stubbornly refused to co-operate with the surgeon's efforts. I bled a lot, everybody swabbed. The frown lines around the eyes over the mask deepened, the pain grew worse and worse. More and more anaesthetic made no difference, not to the breast that is, although I was almost paralysed down the left-hand side for hours afterwards. Nasty clinking, clanking noises. More pain, more difficult to cope with. Relax, breathe properly, relax. Dear God, help me, I can't bear it. Then comfort; the theatre sister, sitting next to me, putting her arms around me, murmuring encouragement, barking and snapping at my tormentors. I love her. Doors opening. 'What the hell's going on in here?'

It's very strange being conscious in an operating theatre. The blunt unsentimentality leads you to expect Alan Alda and his M.A.S.H. unit to burst in at any moment. Of course, nobody expects to be overheard, but once your state of consciousness is revealed everyone gets very chatty.

'Shut up, we've got a local in here.'

'Oh, sorry. Well, let's have a look.' Riffling through my notes. 'I say, you're an acupuncturist. Why didn't you do this anaesthetic yourself?' Dry-mouthed and indignant I couldn't let that go.

'Because your boss wouldn't let me.'

'Ah, well, he's like that. Unimaginative. He's next door actually – I'll have a word with him about this ... It would have been *so* interesting ... I'd have let you. It really would have been interesting ... Wouldn't that have been jolly interesting, sister? ... OK, OK ... I'm going. Look there's a bit of a pile-up outside – how much longer are you going to be?'

The face with the frowning eyes is sweating now. How much more of this can I bear? He's having a pretty hard time as well. Poor soul, maybe he's never done this before. That makes two of us. Finally:

'I think that's about the best I can do. I'll have to put a

11

drain in, I'm afraid it's rather messy.'

Caring very little at this stage what he does I am gratefully wheeled back to the ward. Sister squeezes my hand and kisses me as I leave. I love her more than ever.

They brought me tea in bed.

'Technically you are a day patient, but things didn't go exactly according to plan and we'd like to keep an eye on you, I'm afraid you'll have to stay.'

Working mothers with three young children are easily bought with tea in bed, and I decided to make the best of it.

The consultant was visibly embarrassed at the sight of my wound, not least because the drain was in the wrong place.

'He's put it at the top instead of the bottom, it was because you were lying down I expect. It's not much use up there I'm afraid, we'll have to take the stitches out, then you can drain through the scar. Sorry about this, but it could happen to anyone.'

I'm sure it could, and frequently does, but why me?

Huddled in pain and misery I watched the Bavarian landscape from the window of the train. Exquisite, story-book chalets peeped through the trees and I was expecting Julie Andrews over the hill at any moment, but that was no comfort to me. Even the unbelievable charm of the train stop (one could hardly call it a station) gave me scant pleasure. This was where we made our final connection with the bus for Bad Weissee.

To my annoyance David seemed to be enjoying himself. He admitted sheepishly, 'I've always wanted to see this part of the world.' But even I cheered up a bit on the bus. After all I hadn't actually died on the trolley at Munich station, and we were so nearly there, the chances that I would make it all in one piece were pretty good. Most of all, though, I was excited about meeting Issels.

Among the many threats and promises my doctor had made while dancing with rage around my bed at home, was the assurance that Issels was only after my money, and that he would 'soft-soap' me into staying. My protestations that we had bought short-stay tickets and would make a rational decision based on what we saw and heard cut no ice with him.

'He'll talk you into it, I know he will.'

I freely admit that after the weeks of fear and negativity I was indulging in a little luxurious anticipation of the soft-soaping. Anyone who knows Josef Issels will appreciate the funny side of this.

We arrived at dusk. The RingbergKlinik. Was this really happening to me? An immaculate, efficient, bi-lingual receptionist told us to wait. We waited. Pale, sick people shuffled past, staring sharply to see which one of us it was who had been marked to share in their special community. I could hardly bear to look at them. Had they too once sat here, also imagining that they would recover, that they would never be as sick and ill as the people they saw? The all too familiar tears welled warmly into position, but I struggled hard to contain them. I was hoping my interview with Issels would have the singular distinction of being conducted dry eyed.

David had his eyes closed. He looked pale and exhausted, an even better candidate for the cancer club than I imagined I looked myself.

I remembered what a dear friend of mine had said, when in desperate anguish she had agreed to go to mental hospital, and asked me to take her. Just before the doctor came to interview her she said, 'Let's not tell them which of us is me.' I've often wondered how long it would have taken them to find out their mistake.

Eventually we were led through treatment rooms, mercifully free of the sad, ghost-like patients, to a white-tiled, white-walled, white-floored examination room. All glittering chrome and bright lights. We sat dazzled and blinking. David looked even worse in this light. I told him to watch out or they'd be after him too and we both burst out laughing as Issels came in.

Josef Issels is one of the Giants.

To say he 'came' into the room is not strictly accurate. He is a man who makes entrances and exits. He doesn't 'talk' either, he makes utterances and statements, and he doesn't go in for 'soft-soap'.

He was dressed entirely in white: white trousers, white shirt, white tie, white coat, white shoes and white socks, conveniently topped off with an impressive shock of white hair.

He asked the obvious and familiar questions about my case history and what treatment I had already had. Later he was to refer to his English as, 'Klinik English – no good!' but it was possible to communicate with him from the very beginning.

'We treat everything here, you understand: the whole body, not just the tumour.'

Yes, we understood, we liked the sound of that, that was why we had come. But what did his treatment consist of and how effective was it?

With obvious effort he controlled his impatience. He was tired, he had had a long day and we were getting on his nerves.

'You don't like my ideas, don't stay.'

So much for the soft-soap.

We had come in order to stay a few days and see what was going on, so, as Issels swept off for supper, we tottered up to bed. It's marginal which of us was the more fed up and exhausted.

Next day we tried to work out what the therapy actually involved. All the staff were kind and helpful and gave us as much time and as many explanations as they could, but it is in the nature of multiple, holistic therapies to appear a bit puzzling at first and we were very confused. My uncertainty was exacerbated by the fact that all the patients looked so very sick and ill, and these were the ones who were up and about. Goodness knew how much more suffering was going on behind the bedroom doors.

I was yet to learn that most people turn to less invasive, holistic methods of treating cancer only after they have run the gamut of other, more orthodox, methods. Somebody presenting themselves, untreated, at my early stage was a rarity. It was hard to judge how well things were going for these people because they were, quite simply, either very ill indeed or nearly dying.

There was one other English girl there, Sandra. I think

Sandra was an angel, but if she wasn't, she certainly looked the part. She had the most amazing golden-yellow hair that I have ever seen, but she was crippled with extensive secondaries. In her way she was typical of the patients in the clinic: she had been a cancer patient for a long time and had a long history of surgery and radiotherapy and chemotherapy treatment. She had come to Germany in desperation, having been told that there was nothing more that could be done for her. Quite understandably her commitment to the clinic was one of more faith than judgement, and she and her husband watched with detached interest as David and I conducted our attempt at an objective fact-finding mission.

We had several sessions with Issels. He was desperate to start me on his therapy. I was wasting precious time, he said. The sincerity of his anxiety was palpable, so too his evident certainty of the efficacy of his system, but I remained dogged in my resistance. Not so much as a grain of vitamin C was to pass my lips until I had mapped out some sort of plan. He thought I was mad. There was now a fairly long list of people who thought I was mad; I probably was a bit mad.

The other patients and staff were puzzled. Yes, I did have cancer. No, I wasn't a patient. Why not? Why not indeed. I sought in vain for evidence of crookery and charlatanism, but was anyone likely to leave such evidence lying around, and would I know it if I saw it?

Later that first day, patiently discussing his beliefs and techniques with us, Issels broke off, turned to me and asked:

'Do you know why you've got it?'

It is hard for me to describe how I felt at this moment, it was so powerful and such a significant turning point for me. Here was a doctor who wanted to know if I knew why I was ill, who didn't think that was a peculiar concept, who asked the question in a matter-of-fact way, almost casually.

'Yes! Yes ... well I think I do ... there are lots of things ...'

It occurred to me later that our attempts to be investigative and objective had put Issels somewhat on the defensive and consequently we had cut ourselves off from the line of communication that really mattered to me.

He smiled and said that I must deal with all that. He would work on my body, on the physical side of the problem,

15

but that would be pointless if the psychological and spiritual problems were left untouched. I nearly wept with relief. This was the first discussion I had had with anyone since Diagnosis Day that made any kind of sense to me.

I threw away my return ticket and stayed for nine weeks.

David was able to stay one more night before the expiration of his ticket, returning the following day to rescue our children from their unavoidable separation to different friendly homes.

This was to be a memorable night. My certainty, now absolute, that my tumour would never be overcome except by a total cleansing of myself presented me with a dilemma. Like most married couples, David and I had accumulated our fair share of junk over the years, which we had carefully been brushing under the carpet and assiduously trying to ignore. If I was to justify my decision to stay at the clinic, and spend a fortune of money we could not afford on Issels' attempts to clean up my body, it seemed ridiculous for me not to clear out some of the bigger pieces of lumber that were cluttering up my emotional life.

I had no doubt that this long overdue spring clean was an essential pre-requisite to the course of treatment on which I was about to embark, the dilemma existed only because I was afraid. I was not a person renowned for my courage at the best of times and I feared that this encounter might prove altogether too much for me. If things went wrong I could see myself adding so much more to the burden I was already carrying (a marriage on the rocks for example), that I might be running the risk of falling, literally, at the first fence. Nevertheless I had already journeyed a considerable way down my all-or-nothing route and I felt committed to this course of action, despite a great deal of anxiety and trepidation.

My long-time friend and bridge partner had taught me always to play contracts the only way they could be made and risk going down in an expensive heap if the gamble failed. His equivalent of a bunch of grapes was to send me a rather seedy picture postcard of Leamington Spa bearing the command, 'Remember to play it the only way it makes.' Despite his confusion, shared by most of my friends, over what I was actually up to, he sensed the danger of my dilemma and in his cryptic missive gave me just the advice I wanted to hear. I was going to go for bust.

As it turned out, I need not have feared. David proved to be just as keen as I was to undertake this exposure, and we lay together in the darkness of a strange room in a foreign town and played a grown-up version of the children's game Truth, Dare, Kiss or Promise until way into the night.

Instead of the hours of accusations and recriminations that I had anticipated with such dread, we found ourselves capable of real forgiveness and understanding. I had expected another long run-in with those old favourites, guilt, blame and shame, with all the attendant revenge, martydom and point-scoring so familiar to us all. (Especially familiar to people who have had fifteen years of married life in which to hone their techniques to perfection.) But, this time it was different.

The erstwhile boring predictability of the tenor of our discussions was finally blessedly transcended. We were able to jump off the treadmill of 'But you always . . .' and 'That's because you never . . .'. For once we managed not to justify our own weaknesses and failures on the basis of being married to someone who was even worse.

We started to accept and forgive each other. Borne along by the balm of relief we whispered on and on through the night. Now that we had started we didn't want to stop.

For the first time I saw my husband as a human being with hopes and fears and strengths and weaknesses and blocks and barriers, just like me. I also saw, to my amazement, that most of his negative behaviour came from reacting to me. Having mapped out for myself the role of innocent-victim-driven-in-desperation-to-a-few-small-misdemeanours, it required more than a little effort to entertain the possibility that David's view of me might hold a grain of truth. He had me marked down as an implacably self-righteous martyr, one who gave everybody a hard time because they weren't coming up to expectations that were never made clear and were therefore impossible to fulfil.

Take your pick, dear reader: it's only a question of perspective. 'I'm discriminating, you're fussy; I'm sensitive,

17

you're touchy.' You know the sort of thing.

One way and another we covered a lot of ground that night. We have both, subsequently, worked very hard on ourselves in trans-personal groups and individually, with counsellors, healers and analysts, but I can honestly say that I have never moved so far or learnt so much as I did that night. Talking about this years later to a medical friend he said confidently, 'Oh yes, I can understand that happening, it's the effect of the shock you know.'

It is certainly true that the shock of the diagnosis had forced me into initiating this extraordinary dialogue between David and myself, and maybe its effect on David had been to enable him to drop his critical, hectoring style for a much softer response. After all, you can't give your wife a verbal battering if you think you might not be seeing much more of her. Not only was he listening to what I had to say, he was acknowledging it as well. I had, in a phrase, never had it so good.

I am one of the many people who say they are glad they had cancer. Not being frightened of flying in floppy-winged aircraft was the least of the spin-offs. The indescribable sweetness and joy of that night and the peace that came from it was so beautiful a consequence of being hit by a virtually incurable disease that I can honestly say it was worth it.

Months later I tried to explain to a friend how cathartic and healing the whole experience had been. She said how much she would love to risk such a session with her husband, but simply lacked the courage. 'It was easy for you,' she said wistfully, 'you were lucky because you got cancer.'

Shocked at what she had said, she protested that wasn't what she meant, but of course it was exactly what she meant, and she was right.

By the time the night nurse came in at dawn David and I had tipped out every last bit of rubbish from a great emotional dustbin. We lay exhausted and grateful. Rejoicing in the comfort that comes from being exposed, recognized and accepted. I suppose, despite the depth of our feeling for each other over the years, this was our first tentative offering of unconditional love, and it felt wonderful.

18

Naturally we thought that we had solved all our problems with one fantastic stroke and imagined that from that moment on we would proceed in total harmony and understanding, with lots of laughingly tolerant generosity of spirit swilling all around for the rest of our days. Of course we had done no such thing, but we had hacked a way through the jungle of thorns that had grown up around us and the Sleeping Beauty of our precious marriage was at least awake again. There was a good deal of tidying up to be done in and around the palace grounds, but at least it was possible to get to work.

Having to be parted after this sweet, new experience of each other was agony. Feeling so much closer than we had for years it was terrible to have to leave each other, but there was no question of David staying to support me while we were both so worried about the children.

Daniel was twelve, Justine and Jessica ten and nine. Old enough to have overheard the desperate telephone calls and the tense discussions; old enough to have been told their mother had cancer and old enough to realize that our panicky behaviour belied our confident reassurances. Not, however, old enough to cope very well with their own shock and fear without the help of their parents.

I was deeply conscious of the fact that had I been less rebellious I would have been in hospital at that time, a few miles from home. They could have come to see me, crayoned a few Get Well Soon cards, brought flowers from the garden, and generally enjoyed a much easier time than they were having now. My sudden and uncharacteristic burst of selfish, independent behaviour had caused them all sorts of problems.

So, although I wanted David to stay longer with me, I wanted him to go home much more, and thus it was as the bus pulled him away from me I diverted my misery into picturing how thrilled the children would be to have him back.

With a show of bravado I did not feel I strode back into the clinic and hurled myself into getting well again.

Chapter 2

We must completely rethink our position. We need to go back to the old days when a doctor looked at a patient as a whole. We must seek the cause of an illness. We must combine humoral pathology with cellular pathology. Both are of equal value.

Josef Issels

The aspect of Josef Issels' therapy that distinguished it from anything I had been offered until then was the fact that he treated the whole person and not just the tumour. He referred constantly to 'whole body therapy' and earnestly insisted that, 'You must change the "milieu": you must make it impossible for cancer to grow in your body.'

By the time I finally took up residence in his clinic as a registered patient I felt I had already made a valiant attempt at weeding out the cancer from my mind and I was looking forward to finding out just how he was planning to do the same thing for my body.

I was given a room on the top floor of the building with a picture-postcard view of the mountains. There was a proper hospital bed for me and a sort of divan affair where David slept during his visits. There was one moderately comfortable chair, where I spent an inordinate amount of time in the evenings, and a small desk at the window. I also had an adjoining, private bathroom for which I was to become increasingly grateful.

Since I had not wished to pre-judge my decision about staying longer than four days I had only brought a few things with me and it didn't take me long to unpack. I looked at the pathetically small impression that my being there had made on the impersonal, white presence of the room and wondered tearfully for the thousandth time if I was big enough for the task ahead.

The nurse who was appointed to outline the daily routine to me was selected more for his willingness to try than for any notable command of the English language. Despite this he was a good choice, since his bizarre similarity in physical appearance to Rupert Bear's father endowed him with a comforting aura of avuncular dependability. We spent hours at a time in the treatment room (one on each floor, where all the equipment was kept, injections given and notes filed) while he tried to explain the therapy to me. We ran the gamut of communication techniques, familiar to all those who have tried to exchange information without the advantage of a common language. There was the inevitable tendency on his part to say everything louder and louder until his thundered exhortations became the subject of complaints from resting patients. For my part I found myself encouraging him to repeat things, as if this pointless exercise would somehow result in my lack of understanding being worn away by forceful and constant attrition. But, odd as it may seem, our initial struggles served to endear us quite deeply to each other, and during the subsequent weeks of my stay it was his habit on meeting me anywhere in the building to burst out laughing and scoop me up in a warm and comforting embrace.

When he finally abandoned language in favour of a form of enthusiastic and energetic charades we got on much better. I can see him now doing an exaggerated imitation of someone swallowing tablets: first indicating a running tap, then tossing the required amount of pills into the air and finishing off with an eye-starting gulp and a slap on the chest to help them go down.

There were tablets to suck, there were potions to rub in, there were liquids to be diluted and consumed at regular intervals throughout the day. There were pills to be taken before meals, there were pills to be taken after meals, there were powders to take on days when you didn't take the pills. There were things that had to be done on alternate days, but you had to ignore Sunday. There was a daily chart to be filled out with information about pulse rate and temperature (and all hell was let loose if you made a smudgy mess of it). There was a funny-smelling body rub for right arm, left leg one day and vice versa the next. There was some kind of Star Wars machine in the basement that purported to do something for your glands, and more, much more.

Naturally it had been my intention to have a coherent understanding of every aspect of my treatment; not for me the mindless, unquestioning acceptance of the unknown. But it soon became quite clear that merely establishing *what* I had to do was a mind-blowing task in itself. Comprehending the details of how it was all meant to work would have to come later. It took me days – no weeks – to get the system working smoothly.

In the early days I was for ever arriving just as they closed the short-wave therapy room, taking my 'after' pills 'before' and forgetting to drink my potassium, so having to down pints of it at bedtime, ensuring a most unrestful night. But gradually it all started to fall into place and a pattern slowly emerged.

My friendly Father Bear did his level best to help. He developed a nice line in stick-cartoon-men, and it is to my great sorrow that I no longer have his particularly clever line drawings of how to prepare and administer a coffee enema. However, nothing can erase from my memory his rather startling mimed actions, worthy of a very keen contender on 'What's My Line'. He would undoubtedly have beaten the panel.

It comes as a surprise to most people to hear that, although you are not allowed to drink coffee on any self-respecting holistic cancer regime, you are allowed to do the other thing with it. More than allowed, encouraged, forced almost. The theory is that coffee absorbed through the rectum causes the gall bladder to flush out bile and toxins, thereby refreshing the liver. If this sounds a little bizarre and unlikely I can assure you we all took a bit of persuading as well.

Most of the pills and potions were vitamin and mineral supplements and homoeopathic preparations. There was also an immune stimulant made up from one's own blood, and a self-administered substance described as a vaccine that was also prepared homoeopathically. Getting this lot organized into a workable routine was actually very therapeutic in itself. I wanted to be active in my own defence. I had never warmed to the role of passive recipient in the medical model; this busy involvement was much more my style.

I think it would be fair to say that the main thrust of Issels' approach was immunotherapy. My desperate researches from my bed at home had revealed the existence of this approach and it had appealed to me. My doctor had assured me, 'It doesn't work. Of course it doesn't work. If it worked, we would be doing it.'

Nonsense.

Acupuncture works, but that doesn't mean they teach it in medical schools.

Most of the RingbergKlinik medication was aimed at raising the body's own defences against cancer, rather than mounting a direct assault on the aberrant cells. Although he made use of cytotoxic drugs and radiotherapy in the treatment of some of his patients, Issels' main concern was to reawaken the body's own mechanism for repelling invaders. He only saw these other invasive, destructive treatments as a part of a broader plan.

He was very worried about the state of my breast. I had an enormous haematoma that glowed every colour of the rainbow and oozed alarmingly into my twice daily dressings. He and his colleagues responded to this sight in the time-honoured style of all technicians – builders, plumbers, hairdressers alike – by sucking in their cheeks and shaking their heads in disbelief, wondering how they could possibly do a good job when the person before them had done such a bad one. There was talk of a mastectomy.

This did not fill me with horror. My response here was quite different to the way I had felt in England. There the proferred surgery represented the solution. Here it was only one step on the road back to health; just one of many moves that might help me to get on top of this disease. As such it was a much more acceptable proposition.

Fortunately we all decided to wait a few weeks and see

23

what happened. What happened was that my breast healed up beautifully, and talk of further surgery was soon forgotten.

In addition to the immunotherapy treatment we were all put on to a detoxification programme. After all, if the body does begin to break down the cancer cells, one wants to encourage the dispersal and evacuation of the toxic by-products. The liver, being the main organ of detoxification, came in for a lot of attention. Hence the coffee enemas.

I was horrified by the idea of these enemas and resisted them pretty strongly.

'Look, I'm not very toxic anyway. I've been eating good clean stuff for years, I'm sure I don't need them.'

But nobody listened, because of course I did need them.

Every day I collected my jug of steaming brew and juggled around with it in my bedroom. Such was my resentment and tension, everything that could possibly go wrong went wrong. It was either too hot or too cold, or the gravity tap got stuck and nothing flowed properly, or I felt so uncomfortable I couldn't hold the wretched stuff for more than a minute. I wasted gallons and gallons of coffee and positively enjoyed telling everyone that they didn't work. I had a lot of prejudice to overcome in relation to coffee enemas and it took me a week or more to realize that I was being a bit childish. Once I decided to stop fighting so hard against them, but to try and entertain the idea that they might be good for me, then naturally I mastered them perfectly well and, much against my will, was forced to admit I felt better for them.

In order to encourage detoxification through the skin we were encouraged to give ourselves brisk, dry body rub-downs at the beginning of the day. We used brushes, or gloves knitted out of scratchy, old-fashioned string and kept rubbing till we turned pink. We were then supposed to leave the pores open, not finish off with a cold shower.

One day Issels suggested, 'Go to the hot room in the town. This is very good.'

I managed to establish that he was referring to the public sauna and greeted this suggestion with some cynicism. I felt so weak and feeble I couldn't imagine surviving a sauna

24

without fainting at somebody's feet and decided to save that treat until I could take a friend with me.

Some of the therapy was designed to oxygenate the body. Cancer cells thrive in yeasty conditions and don't like the presence of oxygen, consequently we were all encouraged to exercise as much as possible, or at the very least do deep-breathing routines. Issels is famous for coaxing his patients high up the mountains and leading them through a few breezy oxygenating exercises. He had also devised a way of injecting ozone into the body, intra-muscularly and rather painfully. There was a machine in the treatment room that was used to fill alarmingly large syringes with the required amount of ozone and which, mercifully, kept breaking down, so we were sometimes spared this discomfort while not actually having to refuse it.

However, there was another oxygenating technique, which always worked with dependable efficiency, that I found particularly terrifying. In a basement room that glittered with a reassuringly sterile atmosphere I lay back and allowed someone to open my veins and help themselves to a good supply of my blood. This was then 'oxygenated' by means of a process I can only describe as being 'pretty', because everything was done in a beautiful blue haze, but I cannot offer anything more scientific. This revitalized blood was then returned to me. The frightening part of this sequence was the presence in the treated blood of a great many air bubbles. Indeed, what was eventually fed back into my veins was something that looked like a well-shaken bottle of Coca-Cola, consequently I lay in fear of imminent miocardial infarction or worse and, like many another cancer patient, felt grateful just to have survived the treatment.

Nothing, however, quite equalled the misery of fever days.

Once a week we had to skip breakfast and started the day with an intravenous injection of b-coli virus. This had the double-bonus effect of inducing a massive immune response in the body, stimulating a huge production of white cells, and at the same time ensuring a significant rise in body temperature. The net effect of this was bad news for the cancer cells and none too terrific for the rest of you. I

25

remember the fever days as a blur of pain, nausea, sickness and distress. In between the halucinations and vomiting you were expected to keep a half-hourly record of your pulse and temperature, an almost impossible feat if you were alone. As I was.

A lot of the other patients were there with relatives who could help them and I soon learned to beg anyone kind enough to visit me, please to do so to coincide with a fever day, but initially I had to cope alone. Once, Sandra – the other very sick English girl who was there – lent me her husband Bob to see me through the worst of the day, but otherwise I groaned and sweated my way through without help or comfort.

Issels always looked in on you at least once to check the progress of the fever. Although his style was tough and uncompromising in the normal run of things, I remember his gentleness and kindness during these ordeals. Sitting on my bed, softly touching my sticky, sore face:

'This is good. Wonderful. Such a fever! You are beautiful with this fever.' And as if to prove it, bending down to kiss me. His medical out-riders looking embarrassed and confused in the background.

The thundering speed of my heart and the almost unbearable pain always led me to believe that each fever day would be my last, an opinion I somehow managed to communicate to Issels despite my melting mind and parched lips.

'No, no. The cancer cells, they do not like the heat, they die before you do.'

Such a comfort.

It was the day after a fever therapy that, for the first time, I went to bed during the day. I was feeling very ill and very sorry for myself. Issels burst in:

'Get up! You must get up. Go out and walk.'

I did not receive this well and protested that I would do no such thing. I was ill and I was staying in bed. I was paying an arm and a leg to entitle me to this bed and I was staying in it.

'You must not do this, people die in bed! You must get up.'

Realizing that he was not making the impression he wanted on me he turned to leave.

'Do what you like, you are the one with the cancer, not me.' And so saying he swept out.

I was shattered. As I tottered out of bed and dressed myself shakily I admitted that there was still a lingering part of me that was trying to put someone else in charge of this cancer. Although I had made such a song and dance about it being my crisis and my body I was still tempted, when the going got really tough, to start looking around for someone else to take it on.

I dragged myself out for a walk. He was right: I was the one with the cancer and I was the one who had to fight it.

I may not have been a willing participant in the fever treatment, or any too thrilled with the coffee enemas, but I was a big hit in the dining room. If it had been possible, literally, to eat one's way back to health I could have done it.

By training and instinct I had come to believe that nutrition plays an enormously powerful role in our physical and mental well-being. My mother's attempts to make all of us drink cabbage water during our formative years in pursuit of a positive multitude of mysterious and unrevealed benefits had not, surprisingly, deterred me from developing an interest in natural foods. Consequently, I was much more at home in the dining room than many of my fellow-patients.

The nutritional rules were basically the same for all of us: no animal protein, no poisons (tea, coffee, artificial colourings, preservatives, flavourings, etc.), low fat, no salt, no sugar, and as much raw food as possible.

It would give me a great deal of satisfaction not to say another word about diets for cancer patients. I actually took with me to Germany a book that laid down an appendix of rules and regulations concerning food that made the ten commandments look flexible, and during the time that I was there I collected quite a few more, just as dogmatic and all annoyingly different in one way or another. In subsequent years I have amassed an impressive library of books on this subject and have now reached the stage where I should not be sorry if I never read another line on the matter ever again. The only justification for adding one more word to this overloaded topic is in order to try and simplify the scene a little.

Whereas it is true that there is much to be gained by following a nutritional scheme that has been designed individually and has been detailed down to the last bean-sprout, not everyone can find a therapist sufficiently skilled and experienced to do this. Most cancer patients, if they bother about their diet at all, get their information from books and it is both frightening and frustrating to find contradictions in what they read. If two people, both claiming to be authorities, hold different opinions about the therapeutic value of garlic, does this mean you can or can't have hummus? I arrived in Germany fairly clear about the food side of this cancer business, but became progressively more confused and puzzled the more I read about it.

I remember sitting at my table in the dining room, cautiously peeling an orange that had been given to me with my meal, while reading a fascinating little book about cancer management that stated categorically that citrus fruits should *never* be taken in the first three months. In defiance of the wave of panic that this stirred up in me, I sat slowly and deliberately eating my orange and decided that my way of dealing with all these contradictions would be to stick faithfully to whatever dietary rules people held in common and not to worry too much about the rest.

For some reason no other aspect of holistic therapy attracts as much attention or creates as much confusion as food. This is a pity because it encourages patients who are already anxious to become positively neurotic about esoteric minutiae concerning what they eat. Agonizing about whether or not to eat anything from the deadly nightshade family will seriously affect their mental state, but the ingestion of a few tomatoes is not likely to influence significantly the outcome of their disease.

The kitchens of the RingbergKlinik served food that was faithful to the basic dietary principles, while being somewhat more generous with dairy products than is usual in these places. Issels allowed the use of some delicious goats' cheeses and occasionally we could help ourselves to some Gruyere or Emmenthal, which was a great treat.

Those of us who were considered to be low in protein were

28

encouraged to eat quark for breakfast. For the uninitiated, quark looks and tastes like a sort of cheesy yoghurt, with the merit of being a very acceptable form of protein. It was necessary to eat a surprising amount of this stuff to satisfy the demands of the doctor who analysed the patients' blood and urine samples, and there was a tendency for those of us who appeared regularly on his hit list to try and duck out of sight when his enthusiastic blond head appeared in the mornings. In the case of quark, it is definitely possible to have too much of a good thing.

Otherwise breakfast consisted of porridge, made from a variety of different grains, or an absolutely delicious muesli, which we ate with yoghurt or buttermilk. There was a plentiful supply of beautiful bread full of all sorts of nutty, crunchy bits, but there was not very much to put on it. The small ration of tiny little butter pats reluctantly supplied by the kitchen were used sparingly and consumed guiltily. Sometimes it was possible to have honey, but this required a special trip to the kitchen, and one's reception there was uncertain. Although there were days when these precious little pots were handed over with a generous hand and warm smile, there were other times when the same request was greeted with a torrent of verbal abuse and much angry arm-waving. In all the time that I was there I was never able to ascertain the reason for this idiosyncratic response, but the challenge only added to the sweetness.

Although the other two meals consisted of cooked food, we were expected to eat as much as possible from a wide variety of raw food that was laid out like a buffet from which we helped ourselves. There was always an impressive selection of different vegetables as well as the traditional salad foods, and everything was thoughtfully displayed and decorated. Despite this, I was sometimes the only person who ate more than a token helping of this food.

One of the reasons for this was the fact that I was accustomed to eating this way, but there were other factors in my favour. My cancer had only recently been diagnosed, I had not been ill for long, or suffered the side-effects of any other form of treatment. I was basically strong and enjoyed the full use of my gastro-intestinal tract. I also had a hearty appetite. This could not have been said of many others at the RingbergKlinik.

Sandra, poor girl, was eating pathetically small amounts – not enough to nourish a healthy body, still less one full of greedy tumours. It frightened me to think she might have left all this too late.

Unfortunately, I now know that cancer patients tend to present themselves for holistic therapy only when all else has failed, and most of Issels' patients would have been classified as terminal. These poor souls simply could not cope with the ingestion of large amounts of raw food. It is actually quite hard work to munch your way through mounds of carrots and cabbage, and the windy consequences were painful and uncomfortable for those who had little strength left save to cope with the suffering they already had.

I was also enjoying a more subtle advantage. I did basically understand the principles of whole body therapy and already knew much about the role of nutrition in cancer control. This made it easier for me to cope with a diet that seemed like a cruel deprivation to many of the others. More important still, I had a deep intuitive belief in the value of these methods. I ate the food with enthusiasm and relish because I believed from the heart that it would help to save me.

Very often, just to witness the enthusiastic pursual of the regime by another patient has more impact on the disheartened or the cynical than any amount of so-called scientific evidence. One good case history is worth a dozen scientific studies – to the patient, that is – and it was ironic that I should have started to fill this role almost immediately on my arrival at the RingbergKlinik. I seemed to encourage many of the others, partly because I understood and approved of the system we were all struggling with, but also I think it was quite simply because I was younger and healthier than they were: hardly grounds for proving the validity of the therapy, but so great is the need to have someone in the vanguard showing the way, I was better than nothing. And it has been so ever since.

So, there I was, the model patient. Taking my medication

as per instructions; marching up the mountains and deep breathing all the way; beating the enema kit into submission; writhing my way through the fevers, and finishing up my greens like a good girl. I never cheated in the local coffee shops where many a familiar face from the dining room took refuge. No sneaky food parcels in the wardrobe for me. In fact I was as neurotic and obsessive about the whole business as it was possible to be. Indeed, I was rather offended when Issels, on one of his morning rounds, pounced on a pretty box of stationery, scattering letters and cards all round the room, in the mistaken belief that it contained chocolates. I was playing it the only way it makes, which, sadly, didn't allow for such niceties.

Chapter 3

We do not look at the shadow side of ourselves: therefore there are many people in our civilized society who have lost their shadow altogether ... they are only two-dimensional: they have lost the third dimension, and with it they have usually lost the body.

C.G. Jung

The RingbergKlinik was situated in a small town in western Germany called Bad Weissee. Snuggled between the mountains and the lakeside it enjoyed one of the most beautiful landscapes I have ever known, and once I had settled down in the therapy routine I established the habit of walking for several hours each afternoon. Regardless of what kind of struggle the morning may have been, the afternoons on the mountains released me from the material world of blood tests and injections, drawing me up, literally and spiritually, into a higher world where all was well.

Hour after hour I walked, through the woods and along the paths, sometimes taking a bus to explore a new place, sometimes braving the terrors of the cable-car just for the thrill of flinging my arms out across the valley in a greeting to the unbelievable, distant snow-capped peaks. I did a lot of arm-flinging and leaf-kicking and skipping over pavement cracks because I was making the most of being alone.

There is a world of difference between being alone and being lonely, just as there is between having cancer and being had by it. I kept telling myself that although I had cancer it hadn't got me, and thus, by taking some responsibility for having it, I felt I had some control over it as well. I tried a similar trick with being lonely. Of course there were days when I ached with longing for some real human contact, but at other times I embraced firmly the whole notion of being alone and cut off, and found it had some pleasing and satisfying side benefits.

It seemed as though I had never been alone before. Looking back through the perspective of my life I saw myself as having passed from a childhood – which had consisted largely of an earnest effort to please or achieve in the constant, milling presence of parents or peers – almost without a break into young motherhood and the demands of three children born in the space of three years. Despite the pain of being parted from them there was a liberating joy in being with myself. I talked to myself a lot. Loudly. More than once I heard the approaching conversations of other walkers fade into embarrassed silence as they came towards me, passing this curious, mad Englishwoman with stiff nods and a murmured 'Guten tag'. I didn't care a bit. I had no reputation here to worry about, no status to concern me. For the first time in years I allowed myself not to care what 'other people' thought, and it was strangely releasing.

Releasing it may have been, but was all this jumping into drifts of leaves and talking to myself going to cure me of cancer? I had walked away from treatment based on physical therapy because I was sure I had non-physical sickness to heal as well, and Issels agreed that you had to treat the whole person. But he himself had admitted that his whole body therapy was just that: for the whole body, not the mind and soul. I decided to ask him about this.

'Yes, yes, very important you do these things.'

'What things? How do I know what I'm meant to be doing, and what do I actually do about it once I've discovered what it is?'

'I cannot help you. One time I could help you, in my other Klinik were yoga counsellors – you know the sort of what I mean?'

I knew the sort of what he meant. Or I thought I did. Pity he didn't have them any longer.

Back to the mountains.

When I wasn't talking to myself, I talked to God. I reckoned he had a lot to answer for and I felt close to Him up there, away from any signs of human activity. I knew He was there and I let Him have it. Job was nothing on me. Yes, I was prepared to accept that I had brought this disease on myself through a dimly understood failure to cope with or respond to my life in a healthy way, but why had He made life such a challenge in the first place? And to allow me this heightened awareness about myself without any guidance as to what I should do about it was either capricious or cruel: not very Godlike qualities.

It soon became clear that neither God nor Josef Issels was going to dredge up a latter-day Carl Jung to unravel my knots, so I decided to have a pick at them myself. I changed my tactic from talking to myself, to talking with myself. I asked and I answered and I heard a lot of interesting things. Looking into the dark and painful corners of myself I found a whole huge part of my being that I was keeping locked up and shut away because it didn't cooperate with the personality I was using to present to the world. It was as though the 'I' that I thought I was, and wanted other people to think I was, danced on the worldly stage like a nervous, colourful puppet oblivious to the great, black shadow looming and gyrating behind.

I wanted everyone to think I was confident, kind and clever, while all the time I was also anxious, angry and ignorant. I had made a careful selection of aspects of myself that I believed to be acceptable to others and I had concentrated on those, but I felt the pressure building up from the demons behind the locked doors. Obviously it was time I aired a few of these. But how to do it? Inspired by repeated allegations in various books that cancer patients have difficulty in expressing negative feelings – particularly in their own defence – I decided to start by getting angry.

If I say that I didn't know how to get angry I might give the impression that I was an even-tempered, consistently equable personality, and this would not be true. Like many people who are out of touch with their negative self I never had the luxury of blowing my top, but fizzled away with resentment and irritability instead. Infinitely worse all round, both for me and anyone near me.

Sandra came to the rescue in a most unexpected way. We bumped into each other one day in one of the basement rooms while waiting for a session of negative ionization. This particular treatment was organized by a terrifying square-shaped person, who identified herself as being female by sitting crouched over some embroidery work when she wasn't shouting at the patients. She had on one occasion wrestled from me some tapestry that I had been doing and proceeded to unpick considerable amounts of it, muttering angrily to herself while so doing. This deed had rendered me witless with rage, but, true to form, I had stood by while she did it, and thanked her politely when she had finished.

On this particular day Sandra sensed how sad I was. She leaned her soft, golden head towards me and indicated with an angelic smile that she wanted to say something. I bent over her and she murmured into my ear:

'Don't let the buggers grind you down!'

This was as unexpected as it was funny, and we both burst out laughing.

'It's a proper bugger,' she went on, 'the tumour's a bugger, this place is a bugger and she's the biggest bugger of them all.'

No doubt the idea that Sandra could be crude at all, least of all in reference to her, was as inconceivable to our grim technician as it had been to me, so she greeted our outburst with a cracked smile which served only to encourage a renewed wave of mirth from us.

That afternoon on the mountain I kept thinking about Sandra's insistence that the tumour was a bugger. She didn't think having cancer was in the least bit educational or good for her in any way, as I did. She was cross about it. Maybe I was cross about having it too, but simply not admitting it. Maybe part of me did see the positive side of it, but perhaps I ought to allow another part of me to be angry about it. After all, if I didn't feel angry about having it, then why should it ever go away? I muttered under my breath, 'It's a bugger,' adding nervously, 'Sandra says it's a bugger,' then gaining confidence, beginning to enjoy it, 'It's a bugger, it's a bugger, it's a bugger.'

The mountains reverberated, I stamped my feet, I was really getting into this now. Maybe ruining the tranquillity of the Bavarian countryside was a long way from defending my tapestry from interference, but it was a start. It always feels unnatural when you first get to know feelings you've lost touch with. It seems so contrived, and in a sense it is contrived because you have to make a deliberate attempt to make contact. Becoming so well acquainted with them that these feelings are comfortably incorporated into your life takes time. To begin with you have to practise. Eventually it all starts to come naturally.

I was still at the practising stage when David returned. He tried to understand, but was naturally reluctant to unleash upon himself a dammed-up backlog of resentment from me, and reacted rather warily to my insistence that I should be able to tell him all the things I didn't like about him. I quickly discovered that I could soon put a stop to his attempts to escape from me by shamelessly dragging the life-threatening nature of my situation into everything that passed between us. I watched myself doing this and was amazed at myself, but it was so deliciously effective I couldn't bear to stop doing it.

Imagine an erstwhile weak, ineffective person who cringed and backed away from any kind of force, suddenly finding in her hand a staggeringly powerful weapon that had the effect of vanquishing all comers. That's how I felt. My cancer became a deadly weapon in my hand and I wielded it at the slightest provocation. Having been an artfully manipulative person in the past I now became blatantly manipulative. Thankfully this state of affairs didn't last long. I wanted to be able to deal with things that I saw as assaults on me, but I didn't want to do it by terrifying the opposition into submission. The heady success that came from metaphorically threatening to die when things weren't going my way didn't bring me what I was looking for, but it did give me a taste of what it felt like *not* to be a victim, and I liked how it felt. I felt potent. But I wanted to be able to feel that way without resorting to such cheap tactics.

Anyone who wants to be of the slightest use to cancer patients must understand two things. Not only that there are secondary gains to be had – in the form of getting some attention, being looked after, listened to and so on – but that the patient must learn other ways of achieving these things

36

for himself. Otherwise he will have no option but to continue having cancer, or resort to getting it again.

Despite the fact that I was busy hitting David over the head with my cancerous weapon every time he so much as raised his voice to me, meeting force with force was not what I wanted. I knew from my brief brush with the martial arts that the really powerful way to handle attack was either not to be there at all, or to use the opponent's aggression in order to deflect him. I started to look closely at the implications of these principles.

Once, in my teens, I had so enraged and infuriated my boyfriend that he smashed his clenched fist against the wall, broke two small bones in his hand and was off cricket for months. I was therefore naturally reluctant to investigate what was meant by 'using the opponent's aggression' and decided to work on the principle of getting out of the way.

But how could I 'not be there' when nasty things were coming my way? Obviously by avoiding them. If it was so obvious, why didn't I do more of it? Why did I feel obliged to stand there in the front line and take everything on the chin? Why did I dignify other people's unreasonable behaviour by responding to it at all? After long periods of pushing this question around I was forced to admit that the reason I accepted so much provocation was because I thought I deserved it. The truth was I didn't think much of myself. I fell neatly into the description of the 'typical cancer personality' with a very poor self-image. In short, I didn't defend myself because I didn't think I was worth defending.

I stopped stomping around the mountains shouting 'bugger' and took to reflecting on how to feel better about myself. Since I was short of a few hundred thousand people standing around all telling me how wonderful I was – which was more or less what I wanted – I decided to start the reassuring process myself. My room was now stacked around with piles of books that were pouring in almost daily from friends, acquaintances, former acupuncture patients and so on. They all seemed to be of a self-improving nature advising recourse to all sorts of erstwhile unfamiliar and strange practices, and, valiantly trying to suspend all disbelief, I was steadily and systematically ploughing my way through them

37

all. There was a heavy preponderance of the Do-It-Yourself-Cancer-Cure literature, stiff with appendices and stern lists of do's and don'ts. I was a little wary of all of these. Although it was inspiring to read about people who had escaped triumphantly from grim predictions of imminent demise by munching their way through a field of wheat grass, I held on to the idea that just to copy what someone else had done was to miss the point.

Cancer seems to me to be a most idiosyncratic disease. People with exactly the same clinical diagnosis respond quite differently to identical treatment. No doubt because each cancer is unique to the person who has it. Thus it seemed to me that every patient would need to find his own, individual way through to recovery. Maybe we could help and advise each other, but rigid prescriptions about what to do made me feel uneasy. Maybe every successful cancer cure is like a maze: a path along which one takes a few wrong turnings, has to retrace one's steps from a few blind alleys, and generally feel one's way around before arriving at the healing centre. Maybe too, each maze is different. If we have our own unique puzzle to solve, then taking a detailed map of someone else's is not particularly helpful. We can give each other guidelines, helpful advice and lots of support, but blindly copying each other smacks of the silver bullet theory, and had no appeal to me, then or now.

In amongst the I-Did-it-Myself-Marching-Through-the-Himalayas books there were others of a more general nature. Individual healers propounding their own pet theories and writing about their experiences, with details of case histories. These were absolutely fascinating, but it was hard to contain so many new and bizarre ideas all at once however hard one tried. It seemed that there was something useful in every book I read, but no one book that really said it all. Nevertheless I was certain that there must be one on improving your self-image and I was not wrong.

To my horror the most likely looking candidate was an American publication, redolent with phrases written in capitals or italics for extra emphasis, and positively littered with exclamation marks. I couldn't stand it. Unfortunately I had a feeling that somewhere in amongst this crucifixion of the written word was something I needed. The book was about positive affirmations. I was already keenly in favour of positive affirmations. My mother had introduced me at an early age to the work of Emile Coué and we had marvelled together over his claims to the efficacy of his technique. I believed every word he said, and had many times chanted my way 'little by little, day by day' into 'getting better and better'. Could I perhaps now use similar techniques to revive a belief in myself? The book said you could and explained how you did it.

I asked David what he thought. He had had less time to adjust to the italics and exclamation marks which is perhaps why his guarded, 'Yes dear, I'm sure it's a very good idea' was accompanied by an expression that suggested it was anything but. Not very encouraging, but I was getting used to doing things without outside reassurance and decided to try.

I set aside some time in the morning after the first coffee enema and in the afternoon after my walk to practise what the book told you to do. It all sounded very simple. You just had to relax completely, visualize one of several centres of power in the body and intone the appropriate affirmations.

I found this ridiculously difficult to do. For a start I wasn't sure whether I was completely relaxed or not – and anyway, how completely relaxed could you be if you had one foot braced against the door in case anyone caught you looking so silly, and one eye half open to squint at the book because you kept forgetting what you were meant to be saying? Added to this, I found it surprisingly difficult to visualize. Recalling a childhood full of vivid daydreams that blurred reality with illusion, I expected to be able to create pictures in my mind without any problem, and it was a shock to have to re-learn even this. But the most shocking thing of all was that I couldn't actually verbalize the affirmations.

Lying alone in my room I tried time after time to tell myself that I was full of love and strength and power, but I couldn't. I literally couldn't say the words. My voice was thin and weak and after the first few syllables it dried up completely, leaving me choking on hot tears of mourning. What had I lost? Where was all my inner joy and

39

enlightenment? If I couldn't summon it with my voice, then was it there at all? I was stunned by this experience but it shocked me into a deeper realization that I was indeed out of touch with my higher self, and opening up that communication again became my overriding goal.

Feeling progressively more confident that I was doing the right thing I stuck at my twice daily routine, although it did little initially except to release floods of tears. I copied out the affirmations on to the cards and stuck them round the room; at least I could read them, even if I couldn't say them. But gradually my voice agreed to express what I now so desperately wanted to hear, and in time I grew to enjoy these sessions and felt renewed and strengthened by them.

As the weeks passed I slowly covered the bare walls of my room with all the many cards that people sent, until returning there became a joy and not a challenge. I was literally surrounded by love and kindness and I devoured every sentimental line and every verse that had been chosen for me. Issels thought it was my birthday, 'Congratulations, yes, you are how old today?' The same as I was yesterday, these were just cards from friends because I was ill. 'Then you are much loved. This is good for you.'

It was his habit to visit each one of us every day. In preparation for this we collected our fever and pulse charts from the nurses' room, made sure all the windows were closed and listened out for the sound of the Valkyries sweeping down the corridor. I couldn't work out why all open windows were closed with an irritable bang on his arrival, but Issels had the idea that it was bad for him to move in and out of rooms of varying hotness and was insistent that we should respect this. I did respect this, I thought it was terrific. I was impressed by anyone who had the ability to make his wishes known and have them carried out. I was planning to do a bit of that myself in the near future and the first, brisk footfall outside my door sent me flying to the window.

I always had things I wanted to ask when he came, something that needed explaining, but sometimes he was too impatient to struggle with his 'Klinik English' to attempt more than a couple of sentences before lapsing into swift, unintelligible German with his colleagues. This was absolutely infuriating, of course. They would examine my breasts, axilla and abdomen, scan my charts, evaluate the test results and discuss them hotly for minutes at a time. If I was lucky someone in the group would attempt a stumbled three-word explanation before they all swept on to the next room. I was grateful to Issels, and I was glad to be there, but it did feel as though I was doing it the hard way.

I decided that if I managed to survive this experience I would try to set up something in England where people like myself could pursue a similar course of action.

My next visitor was Pat Pilkington, who sat and listened patiently to my grandiose schemes. I had not known Pat for long, but we were very close and our relationship compensated for its briefness by its depth. She was the most refreshing visitor imaginable. She came laden with goodies: super smelling, frightfully wholesome and organic things to put in the bath, so I could lie in a foot of foam and feel feminine again; some warm clothes to eke out my rather thin four-day wardrobe; the next three books in Anthony Powell's series *A Dance to the Music of Time*, which I rationed to myself as a nightly treat, one I anticipated with exquisite pleasure because it had the capacity of lifting me out of my current, painful obsessions, to join the odious Widmerpool in his totally absorbing world. She was also full of funny stories about things that had happened to her on the journey, and it seemed that every time she left me to rest or get on with my routine, and wandered off into Bad Weissee by herself something extraordinary seemed to happen to her. She would return to my room and recount gleefully tales of being chatted up by eager Bavarians, and we would fall about laughing at how they would have felt if they knew she was married to a Canon of Bristol Cathedral! She was encouraging, loving and supportive and she even nursed me through the beastly fevers.

Surfacing through the black walls of pain I used to focus fuzzily on her figure sitting next to my bed and watch her praying for me. She carried me through many a dreadful day, and I was passionately grateful because I knew what it was like to endure these fevers alone. I was lucky to have survived

41

some of them without serious injury. A young, foolish nurse had once allowed me to go to the lavatory unaided, with the result that I fainted and crashed like a sack of stones on to the floor, injuring my lip and cracking my head, but mercifully not seriously hurting myself. When I regained consciousness I couldn't work out what had happened to me. How had I got to the floor from my bed? And, more to the point, how could I get from the floor to the emergency bell? These were experiences I had no wish to repeat, so Pat's presence was protective as well as healing.

Once the fevers had passed their peak and started to recede, I used to go through a peculiar period of semi-consciousness when I experienced overwhelming feelings of omniscience and understanding. When Pat was there we used to talk our way through these times in great excitement. It seemed as though the storm of my fever had blown away a lot of obscuring clouds and we were able to see ourselves and each other very clearly. They were precious moments. When we weren't sharing our personal insights we were planning what we could do to help cancer patients back home.

As my temperature gradually returned to normal I could serve my raging thirst with weak herb teas, dear Pat standing by lest this should be one of the miserable occasions when it all came vomiting back. It takes a special kind of friend to cope with this and help change the tangled sweaty sheets and help you bathe. Years later, I was to hear her saying on television that she didn't really take seriously all this talk about a cancer centre in England, but was so moved with tenderness towards me that she felt she had to humour me a little. But she too was soon to be taken over by events, returning home from this visit to find a letter recommending a certain Dr Alec Forbes who was interested in new approaches to cancer. Canon and Mrs Pilkington were involved in healing work, would they like to meet Dr Forbes? All this before she'd taken her coat off. Some have greatness thrust upon them whether they want it or not.

I had been in Germany for over a month when the snow came. Issels was furious.

'So much too soon, this is not usual.'

It was indeed early, the beginning of November, and the little town was not really prepared. But none was as ill-prepared as I was, still trying to exist with a handful of clothes suited to a late English summer. I had no proper coat and no shoes. My afternoon walks, which had now taken on the most tremendous significance for me, were threatened. I solved the shoe problem by buying a pair of wellingtons, but even wearing layer upon layer of clothing my light-weight mackintosh was simply not warm enough and the cold was making me miserable. But I could not bear to stay away from the mountains.

I had never seen snow like this before and was enchanted by it. Almost overnight, the puzzle of the six foot poles that lined the higher pathways was revealed. They were markers. The snow was so deep and disorientating that they were necessary to stop walkers falling into drifts, or getting lost. The walking became even more exciting now that it was also tinged with danger.

I was only sorry that there were no six foot high, red and white striped markers showing me the route of my personal path.

Is there anything as strange and transformational as snow? The most familiar scenes are overlaid with mystery and command a new respect. Suddenly nature is in charge again, dictating new rules about where we may or may not safely go. These soft, seemingly innocent flakes, so exquisitely fragile, combining silently and inexorably to create an exciting but potentially, threatening and hostile environment. Children tobogganed with squeals of joy while the local hospital filled up with frostbite and fractures and I hovered somewhere between the two.

I was glad the snow had come early. My father-in-law, desperate to do something positive to help, sent me money to buy a wonderful, warm coat, and the mountains were mine again.

By this time I was pretty well conversant with the metabolic therapy and had worked out an efficient routine for myself. I felt I understood now where all these fevers, injections and blood-juggling sessions were meant to be leading. Sadly, the same could not be said for the intense round of introspection and self-analysis that I was ploughing through at the same time.

Was I entering into this painful arena because I thought it was right in itself, or was I doing it because I thought it would stop me dying of cancer? Most of the time I avoided facing this dilemma directly by telling myself that the two things were inextricably linked together, though deep down I was far from convinced that this was true. If it came to a choice between my immortal soul and a few more earthly years, I was far from certain which I would choose, and I was looking for an excuse not to admit to the possibility that such a dichotomy might exist. But of course it existed. Immortalized in Faust's terrible decision was the ultimate truth that man's real fight is against materialism. While I clung to physical recovery as my goal could I lay claim to be making spiritual progress at the same time?

Obviously it was very difficult for me to shape any of these thoughts into a workable dough without the leaven of a good counsellor, with the result that I tended to ricochet from one extreme position to another. One day I would feel confident that the application of Faith and the acquisition of Grace were all that I wanted, the next I knew that no self-respecting mother would do anything but struggle to stay alive for the sake of her children. Naturally I wanted to do both, save body and soul, but I wasn't sure how to combine these two efforts comfortably without jeopardizing my progress with one or other of them. It was obvious that I had not been able to pursue them both simultaneously in England, otherwise I would still be there. The question that loomed now was whether I was any nearer to being able to do it here in Germany. I wasn't at all sure.

One thing I was sure of was the fact that nobody in England could offer me a cure. Not a sure-fire, cast-iron, guaranteed cure, only a sort of tense, uncertain hopefulness. That was one of the reasons why I had left, and I knew that I would have stayed if there had been any confident promises flashing around, regardless of how mechanistic and ghastly the treatment might have been. Had I therefore been overwhelmed by my emotional and spiritual needs simply because my life was in danger? What a thought.

44

I flirted with the idea of a deal with God: if he would just get rid of the cancer I would promise to carry on diligently with the soul-searching.

I had the feeling He might have heard that one before.

One thing that cheered me up considerably was the fact that I managed to dodge the dentistry and tonsil department. One of Issels' firmly held beliefs is that all foci capable of harbouring low-level infections have to be removed. This automatically included tonsils and any teeth unlucky enough to have root fillings and which were therefore officially dead. For the first time in years I felt grateful at having had my tonsils removed in infancy. Sandra was not so lucky and hers were whipped away under what turned out to be a very meagre local anaesthetic. She had been assured that this was a very minor surgical event, but when I went to see her afterwards she was furious at the casual way in which the operation had been done. It was obvious she was in a lot of pain, and her throat was too sore to allow anything but a short whispered expression of her evident rage. However something happened that distracted us both from details of the operation itself: the glands in her neck went down. Had I not actually seen this for myself I might have found it hard to believe. One day she had significant swelling of nodes in her neck, the next day there was no sign of them.

I was terribly grateful to have neither lymph node involvement nor a set of tonsils to worry about, but I was even more worried about my teeth. My earnest protestations that they were perfectly all right fell on deaf ears. Issels insisted that I should visit their friendly local dentist who would test to see if all my teeth really were alive. He would then report back to the RingbergKlinik. This test involved passing a mild electric current through my fillings and observing whether or not I leapt a foot into the air. Rather like those spiteful tests for witchcraft, the more you suffered the more likely you were to get a good verdict. It was just as well I did. I was feeling pretty rebellious and I would have resisted very strongly any attempts at pulling my teeth. I was under no illusions about this: I could cope with the idea of having cancer but not with the prospect of a toothless grin.

★

So, the weeks went by. Issels flashed in and out banging the windows and muttering over my charts, while I waited for enlightenment to dawn. My initial driving certainty that I knew what I was doing had slowed down.

Why had I struck out for holistic treatment in such a dramatic way? Hardly because it offered the longed-for guarantees; Issels had never come anywhere near doing that. So why, in the absence of his 'yoga counsellors' – the part of his erstwhile therapy that I felt I needed more than anything else – had I chosen to stay and commit myself to his methods?

Although I had no clear answer to this, I think I sensed, like many others who struggle out of the mechanistic model of medicine, that these other methods might be more compatible with my search for mental and spiritual growth. The Bible admonishes us to 'fast and pray' – perhaps it is easier to do them well if you do them both together. Perhaps there was a synergistic relationship here that really mattered.

While I was agonizing over all this I was well aware that the other patients were looking on Issels' therapy in a perfectly straightforward way, as a means to an end. Many of them had been to other clinics besides his and tried other new, untested methods. They used to swop notes about the various places they had been and the things that they had done. They were, literally, 'shopping around' and somehow I found this vaguely offensive. But wasn't that what I was doing? Why was I here and not at home? Because they 'didn't treat me as a whole' – but was the search for holistic therapy just another materialistic grope in another direction?

Confusion.

In a kindly attempt to improve my social life, the dining staff took it upon themselves to seat at my table any guests or patients who could speak English. This was a mixed blessing since mutual language is no guarantee of mutual anything else, but it did encourage me to find out how other people were reacting to the cancer scene. I had already been helped by reflecting on Sandra's response, I was to learn more from other people.

One memorable day I was joined at supper by a remarkably tall, ginger-haired Swedish man. He was called

46

Peter and he was young, appallingly young to be facing a particularly aggressive and invasive form of cancer. Mid-twenties, I think. He had a tendency to shout, so much so I wondered if he might be deaf. He used to lean forward, insisting on close eye contact during our conversations, which was unfortunate in view of his habit of chewing whole garlic cloves to cleanse his blood.

He was aggressively prejudiced against the Germans. Our meals were punctuated by his garrulous complaints against the cooking, the service, the complexion of the waitress, or anything else that he could think of. He voiced frequently, with parade-ground vigour, his surprise that David and I did not also adopt his hectoring style towards our warmongering hosts. Once he discovered that David was Jewish as well as British his astonishment knew no bounds.

'I have heard this about you peoples. I have heard this before that you are not so angry. Why are you not so angry? These Germans, making war and making trouble. And for the Jews, so much suffering. But I have heard this before about you peoples.'

He had also heard, along with tales of The Ugly Duckling and other such unlikely fantasies, that German prisoners of war were treated well in England, and were even accepted into people's homes. Surely this couldn't possibly be true?

We tried to tell him that it was true without upsetting him too much. He was appalled.

'The English are mad.' He would look at us, slowly shaking his head, full of pity, 'mad, quite mad.'

By the most delicious piece of irony I had reached that part of Powell's *Dance to the Music of Time* where a German prisoner is allocated to the family and proceeds to challenge everyone with his bossy, irritable behaviour. Naturally this is greeted with the kind of puzzled tolerance of an equal that is so favoured by the British middle and upper classes, who are not keen to accept that anything out of the ordinary is going on or to get tangled up in anything vulgar. And who, to be fair, would rather try kindness first and see how you go. After all 'fair play' extends to all, even the opposition. I felt unequal to the task of explaining this to my dinner companion. Anyway, I could barely understand it myself

47

and wished to preserve a few shreds of our friendship without challenging him well beyond his capacity to understand my racial peculiarities.

We went shopping together one afternoon and he bought a silly little Tyrolean hat which he perched, ludicrously, on top of his towering, skinny frame and was subsequently never seen without it. This image of him, like an outrageous, Swedish version of Monsieur Hulot is etched deeply into my memory. I hope he came through all right.

He was interested only in the metabolic therapy. It did not seem to me that he was suffering any internal torture or had any intention of doing so. He thought having cancer was just a rotten bit of bad luck, like coming back to the car park and finding that someone had bashed a big dent in your car. He needed mending. That was how he saw his situation, and that was why he was having treatment. He had completed all the usual therapies and had decided to tack this on to the end as a sort of 'belt and braces' precaution. He was not turning the whole thing into an existential crisis.

Although I never imagined that everyone would react to having cancer the way I did, it was nevertheless good for me to absorb the idea that, for a lot of other people, it was just a practical disaster. It slowly dawned on me that hospitals and doctors are more accustomed to looking after people like Peter and Sandra, and I must have come as a rather rude shock. Maybe, just maybe, there was the slimmest possibility that I had been a difficult patient after all. It was many years later before I came to understand just how difficult.

I chewed away at my indigestible dilemma: having marched out of hospital in England because I needed healing in my mind as well as my body, I was far from certain which side I would come down on if faced with a toss up between the two. My hope was that I would never have to choose one or the other, but it seemed to me that most people had decided quite firmly in favour of a single-track, physical approach. I fancied myself as going for broke along a spiritual path, but I still sweated over my blood tests and worried about my X-rays. It was all too apparent that choosing holistic treatment didn't release you from material-istic goals.

During his rounds one morning, Issels announced, 'We have another English here. You can explain him the therapy, yes?'

In this game, anyone who's not in total chaos becomes an expert overnight. Was Issels impressed with my notebooks, diaries and charts, or had Rupert Bear's father burnt himself out as chief explainer of therapies to foreigners and dug his heels in? Mercifully I was to be assisted in this endeavour by a German woman, resident in America, called Marie, who had come back to the RingbergKlinik for a sort of follow-up course. If anything, she was marginally more obsessive about it all than I was and between the two of us we bossed, bamboozled and instructed the new arrival, a vigorous man in his thirties called Tom, in the mysteries and vagaries of the metabolic regime.

His grasp of it was so tenuous, despite our overwhelming effort on his behalf, I dread to think what he would have done if we hadn't been there.

'Hang on a minute, are you telling me that I have to dissolve these tablets in water in this funny looking plastic thing and then absorb them through my backside? You can't be serious!'

'Do you think it matters if you swallow those drops you have to rub in, because I just have. Oh, hell! I suppose that means I must have rubbed in the ones you're meant to swallow. Well, I don't expect that matters much, or does it? Oh God, I'll never get the hang of all this.'

He took to accompanying me on my walks in the afternoon, walking in a sideways scuttle, half turned towards me all the time, and talking.

All the time talking. It was only an overwhelming pity for his almost hysterical panic that enabled me to tolerate this gross intrusion into my soul-searching. It was astonishing to meet someone who was even more frightened than I was.

He had fled to Germany from under the eager, probing fingers of a specialist who wore a wing collar and monocle and expressed a preference for doing his diagnosis 'on the operating table.'

Tom was a squeamish fellow and lacked what it takes to glide under an anaesthetic and wake up wondering how much of you is still there. He ran. He was only under Issels' care because he was too frightened to face surgery. He hadn't the foggiest idea what immunotherapy meant, and cared less. He darted around the clinic like someone on the run from the police, no doubt terrified that He of the Winged Collar would fly out and get him.

Like the rest of us, he took exception to the coffee enemas, but of course we had all the zeal and determination of recent converts, so he could not escape. He trundled off to his room, clutching his kit and an unambitious quantity of coffee, closely followed by Marie who proceeded to shout explicit instructions through his closed bedroom door. Only his frantic protestations that he quite understood what she was saying prevented her from marching in on him and lending a practised hand.

Later that day he approached me after supper.

'Look, I don't quite know how to ask this, but how long are you meant to keep this coffee inside you?'

I explained that thirty minutes was considered ideal, but of course, to begin with, five or ten minutes was pretty good going. He looked amazed.

'But nothing's happened yet!' he hissed. 'I managed to get it in, but I haven't seen it since. Do you think that's serious. I mean, what do you think I should do?'

I must confess I was stuck for an answer, but Marie, choking on ill-concealed mirth, suggested he should simply try again. For several days he battled on, filling himself up with what seemed like gallon after gallon of coffee – all of which disappeared without trace.

Mercifully he was spared any further traumas. As the results of Issels' investigations started coming in it became abundantly clear that he didn't have cancer at all, and he was away on the next plane, but not before I had gleaned a little more understanding.

Talking to Tom had revealed to me a terrified soul. A person positively seething with fear. It was hard to believe that his brief brush with cancer could have been the sole cause of this, and it was just as hard to believe his anxiety would go away for ever now the diagnosis had been repealed. I suspected that all the demons would just be pushed back into the box and the lid banged down on them again. Watching Tom I realized that my cancer had lifted the lid containing all the horrors I couldn't bear to face, just as his had, but, unlike him, I still couldn't quite decide whether to unleash the contents or shove them all back where they came from.

I did have other visitors besides David and Pat while I was in Germany, but understandably they didn't stay long and I spent most of my time alone. I was isolated in every way, as much by my own volition as anything, but conversation with all but a few people was a terrible strain and had to be confined to unsubtle matters. Television was a waste of time and I wouldn't have watched it anyway because it didn't suit my mood, but Sandra's husband, Bob, used to go down to the TV lounge to take in John Cleese striding around Fawlty Towers. He was terribly funny in describing to us the dislocation between the British and German sense of humour. Clearly he enjoyed the audience response, or lack of it, almost as much as the inimitable Cleese. He anticipated with relish the night of the episode concerning German guests at the hotel in which our beloved proprietor goose-steps around the foyer with his finger held horizontally under his nose in imitation of his unwelcome visitors' now infamous leader. To our intense amusement this particular episode was not screened in West Germany ....

There was a small pension in the town where people visiting the RingbergKlinik were often housed, and within a month or two their local choice of taxi driver had escorted enough guests to my door to be well conversant with my condition and foreign status. One day he came to see me.

'Mrs Brohn!' (All the staff used to roll that out with a beautiful heavy confidence, imagining no doubt that it was a German name. In view of the fact that my husband's family were Polish Jews, only a small trickle of whom escaped to the United Kingdom, I felt it more tactful not to explain. When you're staying not a long way from Dachau, the least said the better.)

'Mrs Brohn! There is a man waiting for you.'

'Are you sure? I'm not expecting anyone.'

After all, I never had any casual visitors. People tend to

announce their intentions if they're flying hundreds of miles to see you.

'Yes, yes. Please come now.'

Rather self-consciously I wandered down to the lobby.

There was a middle-aged man standing there clutching a spray of yellow silk roses. He examined me carefully and his eyes widened with disbelief. As I stood trying to work out who he was and what he wanted, he melted into tears, murmuring, 'Only a girl, only a girl ...'

Shaking his head in stunned surprise he thrust the flowers towards me.

'Your friends, I bring your friends to see you. I think you are alone so I take you to see Germany in my car.' His taxi was waiting, engine running, and he took me out for the day.

The roses were dreadful. The sort with plastic stems that you can press the flowers back on to if they fall off. I treasure them to this day. I expect you could quite safely put the whole lot through a hot wash in a machine. They will undoubtedly last for ever, and I'm glad. Really glad. For me they symbolize an act of spontaneous generosity and kindness that I shall never forget. I can see every line of his expression now as his face crumpled with shock and horror when I turned out not to conform to his aging image of what a cancer patient should be. That a complete stranger should break down and weep for me and go so far as to describe me as a 'girl' was so theatrical and wonderful I confess to it adding a special edge of pleasure to my day out. I enthused over every blade of grass he showed me, although, after hours spent investigating local churches and historical landmarks, I returned convinced that Bad Weissee was the prettiest place for miles around.

This opinion was reinforced by a coach trip that David took me on during one of his visits. Our official destination was Oberammergau, but we took a roundabout route and stopped to visit other places on the way. Most memorable was a baroque church that seethed and heaved with such colourful and excessive decoration it was hard to imagine one was in a holy sanctuary. It looked like a fairground and I half expected the wheezy roll of a barrel organ to start up at any moment. The dry dish for holy water was full of flies.

Many of the houses, as well as churches, in Bavaria are decorated with paintings – usually depicting a religious scene. Some of them were really lovely. My history books had told me that Hitler, who came from this part of the world, was a 'house painter' and I had always imagined him slapping on a bit of magnolia emulsion over the wood-engrained paper while hatching up his future plans. All of a sudden the description 'house painter' took on a new significance. Was it possible that his hand had shaped some of these tranquil and enchanting scenes?

It was a disappointingly murky and overcast day. The clouds were low and Oberammergau lay damp and gloomy and unappealing, the shops full of poorly executed, highly priced, woodcarvings. It seemed slightly ridiculous to be there for any reason other than to see the plays.

But a lot of what I was doing seemed 'slightly ridiculous'. It was slightly ridiculous to shout 'Bugger' to the mountains, it was slightly ridiculous to try to meditate with one eye open on the book, it was slightly ridiculous to be the only couple under seventy years of age on the coach trip. Elderly people kept turning around and staring at us as we drove along, wondering what we were doing there, apparently surprised that we hadn't disappeared since they last looked. I began to wish I could disappear. I wished it even harder when we neared Bad Weissee.

David asked the driver to drop us at the RingbergKlinik. I was so angry, I wanted to hit him. Although I had been protected from the responses of the general public to cancer patients by living such a remote existence for so long, I suspected that this label was not one that would pass without comment. How right I was, I was yet to discover, but I had a small taste of what was to come as the entire coachload, including the driver, all turned round, wide-eyed, to get a really good look at me. By the time David returned to his seat next to me I was rigid with rage and shame and horror.

As the bus covered the last few miles I remembered the women who had tip-toed past my bed in hospital, unable to relate normally to me once they knew that I had cancer. I looked at the open curiosity and pity on the faces of the people who had now blatantly adjusted their sitting

53

positions in order to go on staring at me, and I knew that I could not stand much more of this. A role was being forced on me that I simply could not and would not bear.

As the bus drew up outside the clinic I manoeuvered my way down the steps before David and then extended him a solicitous arm. With all the patronizing care that I could muster I pretended to help him walk up the short drive to the clinic entrance, turning to share a few understanding nods with my captivated audience who I was hoping to convince it was he, not me, who was the official resident here. If the role of cancer patient was as unattractive as all that, then I wasn't going to play it.

Apart from a few little breakthroughs like this I had growing doubts about my progress on the psychological, spiritual or mental level (I was never quite sure which front I was operating on), and these fears were soon to be paralleled on the physical front. Despite my model performance I didn't seem to be achieving much. It was evident that Issels had some kind of standard by which he judged his patients' progress and I was apparently falling short of this.

Establishing exactly what was required was roughly the equivalent of pinning down the rules of The Glass Bead game: subtle stuff.

I tried picking a few other brains. Issels had three doctors working with him, two men and a woman. The woman I saw very rarely, I think she was attached to another floor, but she was brought in to examine me from time to time. I rather dreaded this since she was pretty heavy handed: if she examined your axilla you found yourself standing on your toes. The theory was that if she couldn't find anything swelling under your arm, then nothing was. I saw more of the other two and decided to try and ask them how they thought I was getting on.

One was a South American, with a droopy 'viva Zapata' moustache. Popular with some of us because he could be persuaded to part with pain killers during the fevers, but, since they had the effect of bringing the body temperature down as well, not popular with Issels. They often had spirited rows about this.

I had the feeling that he was not a true aficionado of whole body therapy. His advice to me was, 'Go home and have a mastectomy. You should do this.'

He made me swear that I would never tell anyone that he had said this, and departed. I was absolutely stunned. I panicked, of course, cried for hours, rang David, didn't know what to think, went over and over my 'am I here for my body or soul' routine like a hamster in a wheel, before deciding that I wasn't going to take his advice. I had come to hear Issels, not him.

The other doctor was called Klaus. He was a bit perplexed that his name should have the same effect on both Sandra and myself.

'Why do you think it a funny name?' he asked politely.

'No, it isn't funny, it's just that we think all Germans are called Klaus – just like all Frenchmen are called Pierre.'

'But all Germans are not called Klaus ...'

'No, no of course not. Silly of us.'

It was pretty silly, but we needed all the laughs we could get.

Klaus was definitely better value for money. He had a delightfully catholic view of therapy and had once, on a routine ward round, tried to explain something about my clothes – specifically my underclothes. He stood with one of my bras dangling from his finger, his eyes screwed up with the effort of seeking frantically for the right word.

'Silk! Yes silk is good. Not nylon, that is not good. Always silk.'

You can't help but have a special place in your affections for someone who insists on you wearing silk undies.

To be fair, some of Issels' directives were almost as welcome.

'Something more I think is good for you. A little French wine. Very old. Very good. Have one glass each day please.'

Most certainly. This is one prescription I have followed through faithfully. I have an idea of what it's meant to do for my body, but there's no doubt what it does for the morale.

Nevertheless it was Klaus who offered a few words in the direction of my psyche. He turned up in my room one

55

evening unbidden. He had something he wanted to tell me; it was difficult to explain, but he thought it was important. He had been watching me carefully over the weeks and he wanted to help me.

'You try too much. You are too nice. This is from inside you, you must change. I cannot say very well . . .'

He petered out with a grin and a shrug. I must admit I was rather impressed. I'd been slowly coming to this conclusion about myself up on the mountains. Not so much about being nice, but I was certainly trying very hard, and most of the time my trying was to do with being nice.

Clever Klaus. We were frustrated in any attempts to elaborate on this promising start by the dual barriers of language and time, anyway I wasn't ready for any more than a few broad brush strokes. Most helpful of all was the knowledge that he thought these things mattered, and that they were in some way linked with health. Maybe I was on the right lines after all.

On the right lines perhaps, but Issels was not happy about my progress. It seemed that my temperature and pulse chart was not showing a healthy diurnal rhythm and my stoic endurance of the fevers was less productive than before. I was still suffering the same tortures, but my body was not obliging by soaring up to boiling point. This too was regarded as a sinister sign. Despite my best efforts I was not 'doing well'. I was desperate to have a date to go home. I had now long overstayed the original suggestion that I should be there for six weeks and I was aching with longing to see the children. But every time I suggested that I should go home I was greeted with forceful admonitions that my progress did not indicate that I should leave yet. We became increasingly worried about money.

The salaries of polytechnic lecturers, even when combined with those of part-time acupuncturists, do not run to the sort of fees and bills and expenses that I was having to pay. It was only the recent death of both my parents, resulting in my receiving a third share of their modest home and possessions, that had enabled me to come at all. I was running through this legacy at an alarming rate. Soon there would, quite simply, be no more money.

56

Bob and Sandra had packed up and gone. I spent an afternoon with her just before she left when she told me that she thought she would not live very long. All she wanted was to be with her little daughter again, there was no point in staying any longer, she knew her time had nearly come. I went with them to the airport at Munich. Together we struggled with her wheelchair in the lavatory.

'Thank God I won't have to go through all this for much longer,' she murmured, and I tried to hold her in my arms, skinning my hand on the awkward chair.

We sat drinking apple juice, knowing it was the last thing we would ever do together, putting all the love that we had into just being there for each other.

She wished me well with the compassion that is born of suffering, praying that the same burden would not fall on my shoulders, and I wished her a good journey, knowing that her travelling would extend beyond this short flight home. We held each other's eyes as Bob wheeled her away and the crowds came between us. I could still see glimpses of her hair. It was a golden glory to the end. She died a few weeks later.

Other patients were leaving too. Peter had gone back to Sweden clutching an enormous azalea, the size of a small tree, that had been sent to me. I knew I would never be able to take it home myself and I liked the idea of him having it. He bowled away in a little Volkswagen, bent double to avoid crushing his hat.

Marie had gone too. Her response to treatment seemed to have been satisfactory in a way that mine was not, and she departed optimistic and happy.

As the number of people in the dining room visibly dwindled I noticed other changes in the atmosphere of the clinic.

Issels was under pressure from his directors. No longer a law unto himself, he was now vulnerable to the constraints of his financial backers, and they were disenchanted with running a cancer clinic. This kind of therapy worked well for rheumatism as well, and rumours were flying around to the effect that the clinic was going to close down and re-open as a rheumatology clinic, which would make more money and please the local residents.

To my surprise I suddenly became quite decisive. I could continue Issels' metabolic therapy at home, more or less. With the exception of the blood bubbling and ozone injections, which I would be most relieved to abandon, I was doing all the rest myself anyway. I would gear myself up with instructions, buy as much of the medication as I could, and go home.

Almost as soon as I decided to do this workmen arrived and started reorganizing the building. They were literally tearing it down around me. Each day it became increasingly difficult to get in and out of my room. There were sheets draped across corridors, floorboards ripped up all over the place, the sound of drills and hammers tearing through the peaceful atmosphere, and dust everywhere. The day I moved out into the pension, en route for home, they knocked down the wall of the room next to mine. I think I got out just in time.

I had several meetings with Issels to discuss the programme I should follow at home. He was deeply concerned about me and often burst into my room with a few extra tips or words of warning. He had prepared a list of instructions for my doctor, explaining the broad outlines of what the therapy entailed and detailing those parts of it best taken under medical supervision. I was pretty confident that my doctor would cooperate now that the die was cast and he could not be accused of encouraging me in my flight from the more orthodox route. Nevertheless David took a few lessons from the nurses in how to give the injections, just in case.

I said my goodbyes to the mountains and promised to return one day in joy with the children.

Packing up my room was a nightmare. The slow acquisition of possessions over the nine weeks that I had been there now presented me with some difficulties. David staggered over from England with as many empty suitcases as he could carry, but we still ended up struggling with a good twenty carrier bags all bulging with treasures that I couldn't bear to leave behind. The yellow roses for a start. I also had a small private library to transport.

The situation was exacerbated by my last minute, enthusiastic, purchase of a toboggan for my son. This lay in the corner of my room growing bigger every time I looked at it. David showed an unprecedented tolerance and did not point out that I could have bought him a pen knife or a cuckoo clock. By the time we finally clambered aboard my good friend's taxi we looked like refugees fleeing an approaching army. Only a couple of live chickens on the roof could have enhanced that impression.

Issels came to say goodbye. He went over and over what he had taught me. He knew that his was a unique, personal therapy that very few other people understood. He knew better than I did that I would be on my own. One of the last things he said to me was, 'Remember, your doctor cannot help you!'

I was to recall this absolutely chilling remark many times in the future. Issels, who had fought many a round with closed, orthodox minds, knew how impossibly difficult it was for the conventionally trained doctor to open up to new ideas. He did not make this remark either viciously or bitterly. He merely stated it as a fact. I remember him as a Giant because he had the courage to stand up for what he believed in, in the face of punitive opposition. He was a survivor. He had withstood a good deal during the course of his colourful career: the derision of his peers, vilification from all quarters, to say nothing of a charge of manslaughter. He was a man who knew that the tumour was only a symptom of the disease and not the disease itself, and held on to this view when it was not shared, as it is now, by anybody else. He had the courage to try new ideas, and the even greater courage required to abandon them if they didn't seem fruitful. He cared more about his patients than his image. He was emotional and passionate and I shall be grateful to him for as long as I live.

I write about him in the past tense because I have not seen him since, but he is still all of these things. He survived the closure of the second RingbergKlinik just as he had the first, and is pursuing the cause of cancer patients to this day.

He embraced me and we parted.

As the taxi pulled away I felt a terrible sense of loss. He was a marvellous person to have batting for your side.

However, I had other things to think about now. For example, how was I going to get enough luggage for a travelling circus on to the plane without paying a fortune in excess baggage charges? I toyed with the idea of shuffling pathetically up to the Lufthansa desk and murmuring 'RingbergKlinik' in the hope that this would melt reason into pity, but such a course is forbidden if you have opted not to play the cancer patient role.

I need not have worried. The most helpful, kindly, uncritical soul ever to be employed by any airline anywhere, calmly loaded every single thing on to the baggage track without comment: bundles of books tied up with string, a full-size reproduction of Monet's poppy field, dozens of bulging bags, and of course the beautiful toboggan were all labelled and swept away.

The wings didn't flap once all the way back, but I wouldn't have cared if they had.

Chapter 4

Your friend is your needs answered
Kahlil Gibran

We were met at London airport by David's parents. My encounter with my father-in-law was made all the more poignant by the fact that he had started a renewed battle with Hodgkin's disease at precisely the time that I had been in hospital having the dreadful lump biopsy. He had been through a lot since I had seen him and I was shocked at his haggard appearance. He looked pale and thin and awfully ill. We sat having refreshments. He kept looking at me and blinking a lot. The sight of me was making him cry. I took this to be relief and pleasure at seeing me again, but of course he was as shocked by my appearance as I was by his. I honestly thought I looked terrific. I was pretty fit from all the walking, and although I had lost weight, I rather fancied myself a few sizes smaller and thought I cut quite a dash in my new coat. I chattered on about how well I felt, while he took David to one side to say how ill he thought I looked.

I adored my father-in-law. After a very sticky start – brought about by the fact that he wanted his son to marry a nice Jewish girl and not some unexpected Christian shiksa like me – we had forged a deep bond over the years. His struggle with Hodgkin's disease and my confrontation with breast cancer served to draw us closer together than ever. Promising to see each other again soon, they returned to their London home and we set out in the car for our old Georgian house in a village near Bath.

With every mile that passed I grew more and more nervous. Would I be able to run the house properly? I had

61

been spoiled rotten over the last couple of months, would I be able to cope? What about the children? How could I maintain that I was recovering if I still had to have lots of treatment? Would it be possible to protect them from that side of things?

David settled me at home and went to fetch them. I heard them scuttling up the steps, 'Me first, I want to be first!' And then bursting in, only to stop, rooted, in the doorway. They were not sure of me. However painful it had been for them to do it, they had adjusted to another reality, and they were suddenly surprised out of it. They approached me shyly and kissed me carefully: it was going to take a while to readjust. Later they told me that they too were shocked at how thin and pale I looked, and feared to fling themselves at me for fear of hurting me.

Over the next few weeks each one of them developed a minor ailment of some sort: a sort throat, a tummy upset, just enough to justify a day or so away from school and at home with me. They did this in a nice tidy rotation, so we were able to mend in private some of the hurt and pain that our parting had caused and regain the closeness that we needed. Children are indeed resilient, but they need to be. They suffer out of all proportion to their innocence.

Daniel told me of a biology class in which cancer was discussed in blind oblivion to his predicament, leaving him in turmoil and in lonely tears in the playground.

Justine described how schoolfriends clamped their hands over their mouths in horror on hearing what had happened to her mother, 'Cancer! Oh how terrible. My Gran had cancer and she died.'

Jessica lay awake night after night thinking I had died. That would explain her father's anguished face and distracted state. Maybe he just couldn't bear to tell them what had happened.

It took us a long time as a family to heal all this.

Now that I was back in my own community, amongst people I knew, I began to experience some of the peculiarities of society's response to cancer patients. Responses not reserved exclusively for us of course: anyone with a really big crisis on their hands can expect much the same, in common with the physically handicapped and the bereaved.

Some people stick faithfully to the scapegoat ritual and put as much distance between them and you as possible. This group contains the friends and acquaintances who would normally have rung up for a chat, popped in for a coffee or called in on their way back from the shops. All of a sudden they don't do any of these things. It also explains the people who would erstwhile have greeted you with a hug and a kiss, now standing frozen to the spot a few feet away from you, blushing and stammering.

There's another group of people who don't exclude you altogether, but who include you in a way that marks you indelibly as the odd one out. These are the ones who, in a perfectly ordinary tone of voice, ask someone standing next to you how things are going, but feel obliged when they turn to you to narrow their eyes in conspiratorial pity, lower their voice to a whisper, and accompany the same question with a slow shake of the head.

Mercifully I was spared the worst.

My rector's wife, herself a marvellous example of how to have cancer and stay truly on top of it, came to see me. In an attempt to prepare me for some of this, and spare me as much as possible, she sat and regaled me with tales of things that had happened to her, finishing up with a description of a one time close colleague:

'She was coming down the road towards me and I was looking forward to seeing her, but she pretended not to see me and crossed over to the other side of the road so she wouldn't have to talk to me.'

Very biblical.

Thank God, nobody actually did that to me, but I soon came to realize that people will go to almost any lengths to protect themselves. It dawned on me after one particular encounter that people might need to protect themselves more from me than from most.

A village acquaintance, a woman I had known vaguely but not closely for years, invited me to visit her. She had heard that I had been 'poorly' and was eager for details. She expressed her concern and sympathy about this, and then added, 'I heard about your father's death, such a pity, he was a lovely man. How is your mother coping?'

I told her that, far from coping, my mother had died in my arms only a few weeks after my father. I found myself scrambling through this as if it was somehow vulgar and excessive to have two parents die on you so suddenly and unexpectedly. It was obvious from my hostess's response that she felt as shocked as Lady Bracknell. I had to make an effort to stop myself from apologizing. Eliot is right, 'human kind cannot bear very much reality.'

It was probably all right to have cancer and lose one parent, or to lose two parents and not have cancer, but I seemed to be piling it on a bit. Sometimes I felt like Richard III and wondered if dogs might bark as I passed.

Cancer seems to evoke in the average man much the same emotions as it does in the people who have it: disgust, guilt, grief and of course, that good old favourite, fear. Just because I was making rather an untidy attempt to grasp this particular bunch of nettles didn't mean that other people intended to do the same. I understand it now, but I didn't understand it then. Just when I needed a lot of support and affection I had to cope with projected fear and rejection, which was hard.

Harder still was getting my self-help show on the road.

I presented myself to my doctor, hoping that he would have shrugged off his annoyance at my burst of individualism, and settle to treating me with tolerance if not understanding.

Wrong.

I sat clutching all my letters and papers and documents from Germany and felt my confidence dribble away with every deep sigh and raised eyebrow they provoked as he read them. Why, oh why did I so desperately need this man's approval? What wobbly little schoolgirl still lived in me that dissolved before the withdrawal of authoritarian rewards?

'I can't possibly do this. I don't know what half these things are anyway. You know that this man and his methods have been investigated and as far as the medical profession is concerned this kind of thing just isn't on. Look, my sincere advice to you is to have a mastectomy, it isn't too late.'

'But my breast is all right now. It's feeling good; even the lumpy bits round the scar are softening up.'

'I'm sorry to say this, but that doesn't mean a thing. Most women who have one lump usually have others in the same breast that haven't made themselves felt yet. If you persist in this course of action you're likely to get a local recurrence.'

Of all the things he ever said to me this last remark was the most potent. It pressed itself deeply into my consciousness and proceeded to haunt me for years. I had absolutely no way of dealing with this kind of negative programming, so I took it on board. I simply didn't know what else to do. It was a statement that fell on me with voodoo-like power and I didn't know how to disentangle myself from its prophetic force.

For weeks I continued to make fruitless attempts to win my doctor over. I couldn't bear to part with him altogether, so great was my need to feel there was someone I could turn to, but each encounter was progressively more draining and depressing. He was so deeply convinced that what I was doing was wrong that I even felt at times that my getting worse would be the proof that he needed that he had been right all along. I don't want to suggest that he thought this consciously, but I knew that he did not expect me to get better. I could just about cope with my own uncertainty about this, but I wasn't strong enough to carry his as well. We struggled on: I was trying to manoeuvre him into saying something positive and hopeful that I could hang on to, just as he was determined to paint the picture as black as possible in order to deter me from my course of action.

I knew no more about the resolution of confrontation than I did about overcoming negative programming, so all my attempts at creating some kind of meaningful relationship with him were doomed from the start. He suggested I should change my doctor. He was, however, unable to resist adding, 'Mind you, I don't think any of the other doctors round here would take you on.'

The only satisfactory aspect of the whole thing was that I suspected I was a bigger thorn in his flesh than he in mine. There seemed no point in changing my doctor, I didn't imagine anyone else would be any different.

Instead I turned to David. He had a pretty steady hand with the injections and rather nervously we started to set up the programme at home. The real stumbling block was the fevers. Issels had been particularly insistent that I should continue with these, but they were an awful challenge. Poor though the nursing presence had been in Germany, it was nevertheless possible for me to call for assistance, and there were people around who would know what to do if things got out of hand. Also, the fever was induced by an intravenous injection that my doctor felt he could not give me. It was one thing for David to boast of his skills with subcutaneous and intramuscular shots, but I had a vague idea it was actually illegal for him to go poking around in my veins with poisons – dead ones or not.

We had no choice.

Once a week we set aside a day and I sweated it out. It was much worse at home. I knew I couldn't call my doctor and even the friends who were not busy ignoring me were understandably alarmed at the prospect of taking part in something so unorthodox and potentially dangerous. Poor souls, they all wanted to help, but I was cutting them off from all the usual channels: they couldn't bring chocolates, offer to come with me for hospital visits, show an interest in results of check-ups. They were hard put to understand, even at the most basic level, just exactly what I was up to. It was difficult for me to explain because, not only did the physical therapy entail an altogether different philosophy, but I was unable to dissociate my whole body therapy from my attempts to get my head together as well. Consequently anyone who showed the slightest interest in me was likely to be treated to an enormous emotional outburst that must have been very hard to handle let alone understand.

There were times when I felt quite sorry for my friends. After all I was damaging the infrastructure of our shared belief system with my bizarre behaviour. Many of them did not approve of what I was doing and it was hard for them to set these feelings aside when relating to me. It's frightening how much we rely on shared opinions and mutually held beliefs to keep a friendship going. Although we would be reluctant to admit it, it is very often the case that when we say

'I really like so-and-so' what we mean is 'so-and-so thinks like me and agrees with me, and I like that'. Those friends who thought my behaviour rash and foolhardy were torn between my need for support and encouragement and their own need to maintain the integrity of their beliefs. They were reluctant to be too interested or enthusiastic about my diets, meditations or any other mysterious remedies they had never heard of, for fear this would consolidate my determination to avoid hospital treatments that they thought would be much better for me. Much the same dilemma as my doctor was having.

Sometimes it was even more subtle than that. A special friend of twenty-five years standing, who could cope with any uncertainty she may have had about the therapy side of things, found my ideas about why I was ill quite impossible to swallow.

'You make it sound as though the cancer is a kind of punishment Pen, I can't believe that.'

'No, I don't think that exactly. I think it might be a consequence of certain things, that's quite different.'

'Well, it sounds dangerously medieval to me. I don't understand it.'

But she tried. Suggesting a meal together. First finding a restaurant that served an acceptable menu, then letting me bounce my ideas and thoughts off her, accomodating my need for acknowledgement with meaningful nods and murmurs. She never let her view of the situation get in my way. She loved me enough to leave her own place and join me in mine – 'dangerously medieval' or not. This can't have been easy to do, but nothing about being a friend of mine could have been easy at that time.

The fact that I was not 'seeing the doctor' or 'under the hospital' meant that the burden of my cancer was not being carried by anyone officially designated to take it on. I kept saying that it was my responsibility, but one look at me was enough to show that I was finding it heavy going. My friends were understandably nervous they might be next in line for having to cope with it. I was hideously demanding of my friends; it's a miracle I still have any.

What I didn't know then was that I was also hideously

67

demanding of my doctor, but that kind of insight takes time.

I had lunch with a friend, himself a doctor in Wales.

'I was furious when I heard what you'd done you know. Absolutely furious, but I've got over it now.'

I was so glad he'd got over it, but I could afford to be tolerant. He was paying for lunch. He was also showing an interest in what I was doing and (amazing!) he didn't feel obliged to point out the error of my ways. He knew I was dead set on my path and there would be no deflecting me from it, so he opted to encourage me. Just what I thought my own doctor might have done.

'Oh no, he couldn't do that. You're a terribly threatening patient.'

'Me, threatening! How can you say that? I mean, just how threatening can you be if you're sniffing and snivelling all over the surgery; grovelling around trying to pick up a few scraps of encouragement. He keeps telling me I'm throwing my life away and you say *I'm* threatening *him*. Oh, come on!'

'You know perfectly well what I mean. You're threatening everything he's ever believed in, everything he's been taught. If you're right about cancer being a disease of the whole person relatively unaffected by physical therapy, where does that put all his hospital training? Come to that, where does it put all the other patients he's sent down that route over the years? You're not just insulting him by not doing what he says, you're threatening his profession and the whole belief system of the organization he works for. I'm not surprised he isn't nice to you. He's probably even more angry with you than he lets on. Probably showing remarkable constraint if you look at it that way. I should hate it if you turned up in my surgery. Very challenging.'

This was all very illuminating. It wasn't that I hadn't thought of it before, it was just that I imagined doctors to be above that sort of thing. Like most people I had rather hallowed the medical profession, endowing its members with all sorts of strengths and virtues that in reality they possess in no greater measure than anybody else. I had, quite simply, expected doctors to be different. I knew that Hamlet and the rest of us were, '. . . indifferent honest . . . very proud . . . revengeful . . . ambitious . . .' etc, etc. For some reason

I had imagined doctors didn't share in this. I expected a few years medical training to have expunged my doctor's ego, leaving him able to relate comfortably to me from the heart. Sadly, they don't teach them that at medical school, so people like me can dance a jig on their desks and not get what they need. Mercifully, attitudes are changing very fast. Perhaps we can look forward to a time when disease is not automatically regarded as a disastrous intruder that must be violently assaulted. Maybe those of us who want to work with it at different levels will find doctors able and willing to help.

My problem at the time was that some of the methods I was using to get to grips with things were unbelievably violent and aggressive. I used to spend a couple of days recovering from the fevers and another three dreading the next one. But I was still unable to tell the difference between paying a reasonable degree of attention to my body's physical needs and knowing when the preoccupation with this was distracting me from healing other parts of myself.

One of my reasons for leaving Germany, despite Issels' insistance that I should stay longer, was my need for non-medical help. It was all very well identifying weaknesses and fears in myself, I had to do something about them. It was lovely to be able to explain to David how I felt, but why did I have to make him modify and adapt his behaviour, when really, I wanted to gain some control over my own? It was easier to tell him what not to do than it was to tell myself what to do. He had told me once that I would force the whole world to shift 359 degrees on its axis rather than change my position so much as one degree if by so doing I had to expose my own weaknesses. I hated him for that, but only because he was right.

Knowing what the problem is may well be a step in the right direction, it may even be a big step, and, having taken it you find yourself with a refreshing new perspective, but not necessarily any nearer to resolving anything.

It was incredible to me that, having realized I needed to be more forceful in my own defence and having become an expert in the use of bad language, I still wasn't finding it any easier to say 'no' to anyone. David took the telephone from me one afternoon, unable to watch any longer as I squirmed around saying 'yes' and meaning 'no' to a friend who wanted something, and, covering the receiver with his hand said, 'Tell her "*no*"! Just do it. Nothing will happen. You've got to do it sometime, do it now. Stop messing about. How's she meant to know how you feel if you don't tell her? Say "no".'

He put the telephone back in my hand and stood next to me mouthing 'no, no, no.' From my point of view it was a repeat of the positive affirmations performance; I seemed to lose my voice, and – unbelievably – blushed red and hot. But I managed it, in a miserable little whisper I mumbled something about 'another time' and went weak at the knees.

It was this pathetic specimen that presented itself to Maxwell Cade for a course in bio-feedback. Thanks to the imaginative promotion of washing powder, I travelled half-fare to London and presented myself at a terraced house in Hampstead. I picked my way downstairs to a small basement room, already occupied by half a dozen or so other people, and squeezed into my place around a table overflowing with various electrical devices. Max's wife, Isobel, who was as warm, chatty and outgoing as he was withdrawn and taciturn, encouraged us to introduce ourselves to each other and say what we hoped to get out of the course. Since I hadn't the faintest idea what I thought would get out of it, this suggestion filled me with alarm. I sat and listened to voices explaining how they wanted to be a better yoga teacher, give up smoking, or pass a dull Tuesday afternoon – at least that's how it sounded to me. As each person trailed to a halt, my heart beat a little faster in anticipation of what I was going to say.

What *was* I going to say, for goodness' sake? I was there because I had got cancer, but was I there in an attempt to cure it, learn to live with it, or die gratefully of it? I was none too sure. I don't know what I said, but whatever it was went down like a lead balloon. I was an embarrassment. My little group didn't know how to deal with me, but why should they? Nobody else did. I dreaded having to face them week after week, but I had reckoned without the inimitable Isobel. Bustling around, busying herself with names and addresses and other trivia, she managed to soothe and reassure

70

everyone and somehow imply that it was rather clever of me to have cancer. If she was an advertisement for bio-feedback training, then I was on to a good thing.

Max and Isobel were consistently friendly and encouraging.
'We can teach you to relax into "a healing state". That's a deep level of consciousness where we believe the body is free to put right whatever ails it.'
To this end I was wired up to a 'mind mirror' and my education began. I watched a screen flashing out the rhythms of my brain and saw how they changed in response to my degree of relaxation, how they were influenced by what I thought.
'It's not only your brain that's affected by these things,' Max told me while fiddling about with a funny little black box that was attached to something he was strapping on to my hand. 'All sorts of things are influenced, your blood pressure, heart rate, cortisone output. You can learn to control all these things. Once you know how it feels to be truly relaxed you will be able to sit back and let your body heal itself.'
It sounded promising. I had only one problem, the Skin Resistance Meter wasn't working. Switched on, with the power turned up full it didn't register at all. Max was telling everyone to set their needles to the middle of the dial on the box, but mine was stuck flat in the corner, not showing any inclination to go anywhere. Most electronic devices that won't work seem to respond to a good clout, so I banged the box on the table. Still, nothing happened. Even a sneaky, damp blow on the metal contacts against my palm and squeezing my hand tight didn't make any difference.
Everybody else had needles flying all over the place, what was the matter with mine? Max checked the machine. It was working all right, it was me that wasn't working. Picking his way with great care, knowing that I was fearfully hanging on to every word he said, he tried to explain.
'Sometimes this happens when people are tired or ill. Their resistence is low and the body is sluggish.'
Sluggish! Mine didn't seem to be there at all. Why did I have to be different from everybody else? I was frustrated and

71

fed up and frightened before we had even started. I already felt a failure and we hadn't done anything yet.

While Max talked everybody through an exercise designed to help people calm down the stressed reaction of their needles, my task was just to get mine moving at all. It was only the comforting flicker of the mind mirror that convinced me I wasn't dead already.

After such a disappointing start it is surprising perhaps that I should have come away from my first class with such a strong sense of well-being. But as I found my way through the rain to Paddington I felt a calm relief settle over me. I knew I was doing the right thing. Everything Max said sounded an answering echo in me. Although my logical self insisted this wasn't going to help – they were just a bunch of cranks in a basement and I couldn't even get the wretched machine to work – my intuitive self told me something quite different. Every Tuesday for weeks and weeks I returned to the womb-like basement and sat entranced, listening to Max and experiencing myself. I was beginning to expand my boundaries.

I bought a Skin Resistance Meter and proceeded to practise various exercises at home with the same manic vigour that I was doing everything else.

I became an even bigger cancer bore than I was already. Complaining that having cancer isolated you from society and it was all their fault, I adopted a lifestyle that was absolutely guaranteed to make me an outcast. I was so busy meditating and visualizing and having coffee enemas and tearing up and down to Paddington on the 125 and trying to make people understand me, I hardly had a moment left for any social life. Anyway, I was so fussy about what I ate I couldn't risk letting a morsel pass my lips that had not been prepared to my exacting standards and thus ruled out the sort of casual entertaining that I used to love.

One of my friends – herself a cordon bleu cook – swallowed all the frustration that my demands created and consistently produced meals according to my specifications. The evenings we spent at her home were a refreshing oasis in our lives. Her husband ate lentils and bean-sprouts as though he never had liked steak au poivre anyway, and they served the whole, organic offering on their best plates with such style and such wonderful wines that I remember those evenings more clearly than time I spent with them last week. It was acts of love like this that prevented me from locking myself up completely.

This was a strange and difficult period for David and me. We felt lonely and isolated by what we were doing and at the same time we were by no means sure what it was exactly that we *were* doing. We were on some kind of personal journey, that was definite, and I was trying to save myself from a potentially lethal disease, but as to the relationship between those two things, that was more than a trifle muddled. Although I had a fairly coherent understanding of the principles of whole body therapy there didn't seem to be anyone around who had seen it in action and therefore I only had my own reassurance that it would actually work. Issels had been right: my doctor couldn't help me, and, as far as I could see, neither could anybody else. Understanding and support were scrappy and thin on the ground. Certainly I could find people who thought that diet might be important and who were supportive and encouraging about that, but they had probably never heard of half the other things I was up to. Similarly, people who understood why I was bothering with the bio-feedback couldn't see the point of the fevers. I sought in vain for somebody who could make sense of the whole.

Meanwhile the fireworks of my own personal psycho-drama were still going off in the background. I wasn't too sure how public a display I wanted to make of all this, consequently David and I spent long hours trying to unravel the tangles between us. This put quite a strain on our relationship since it was not always easy to slip from the role of lover to counsellor to friend as the need arose. We had taken a big step towards understanding each other better during our memorable all-night session in Germany, but it was agonizingly difficult not to fall back into old and painful patterns of behaviour now that the situation was neither as threatening or as frightening as it had been then. The more it appeared that I might be recovering, the more David felt inclined to drop his Student Prince routine for something he found more familiar and comfortable. I was so convinced that I needed to break out of the restrictions that I had surrounded myself with in the past that I resisted this pretty forcefully. I was determined not to use the cancer as a weapon for keeping David in line, but there is no doubt that I had an unfair advantage during the endless soul-searching that went on.

Fortunately we didn't confine our efforts to working out what was going on between the two of us, but spread the net to include other significant relationships that were currently, or had previously, given us trouble. Naturally this was a whole lot easier since we were able to exercise a little more detachment in those areas than we could in relation to each other, but insights gained in this way proved helpful when we turned to face the intricacies of our own relationship again. This also helped us to see that most of our problems came from within, rather than without; from ourselves, not from others.

Slowly we gained more real understanding. As the months went by we realized that the rewards for this kind of introspection are considerable. I was happier than I had been for years. We both were. Since it was so brutally true that we would not have experienced this inner contentment and security were it not for the challenge of the cancer I was more conscious than ever that I was actually glad it had happened.

I also knew that it might easily have destroyed us. We were working at the limits of our tolerance, having to deal with aspects of ourselves that we would never have chosen to face, and this was hard on us both. The cancer, with its implicit threat of death, was forcing us to deal with the unfinished business that usually gets clumped together at the end of the marriage agenda, turning up, as like as not, when there's no time left to deal with it. Knowing that we couldn't assume anything about the time available to us, we were trying to get on with this now. In short we were trying to create the kind of relationship with each other that would withstand the impact of death. I wanted to feel free to die without guilt about my shortcomings as a wife, and David had to feel able to let me die without blaming himself for his performance as a husband. We were trying to get it right now, not in some mythical future that might never come.

Gradually we began to experience the benefits of trying to do this. We were growing stronger, and as we grew stronger we grew braver and risked a bit more. Nothing was easy, but then we were doing it the hard way, more or less on our own. Some of the talks we had were as painful as crawling over broken glass. That, and the thought that I might expire during the next fever, left us feeling pretty fragile. But I needed to pursue all this because I had come to the realization that much of my fear of having cancer was wrapped up in the question of unfinished business.

I often used to wonder why I had been so frantic with fear and anxiety when I first knew how ill I was. After all, with my spiritual beliefs, I wasn't afraid of being dead, and although I didn't fancy the actual process of dying it hardly seemed to justify all the emotion that had been roused in me.

During this time of inner reflection and consolidation with David I began to see that the real truth about my fear of dying had a lot to do with him and the children. In common with many other people I had a personal model of what Wonderful Wives and Marvellous Mothers were like, but I was still in the rehearsal stage, I hadn't quite made mine a star performance yet, so I simply wasn't ready to die. I didn't yet have enough stability or security in my roles as wife and mother to be ready to relinquish them. There was too much left to be done, too much that was unfinished. Spending time picking the bones out of this little lot was well worth while. It took a lot of the fear out of having cancer.

Naturally I had no intention of dying for a while yet and continued with my frenzied round of therapies. I had now given up fantasizing about meeting someone who had done it all before and would hold my hand and guide me through. The more eclectic my performance, the more unlikely this became. I decided to put my energies into sharing what I had learned. To this end I met up regularly with Pat Pilkington to talk about the possibility of setting up a centre in Bristol for cancer patients.

Chapter 5

Either I will find a way, or I will make one
Sir Philip Sydney

It turned out that Alec Forbes was very keen. Frustrated by the limitations of hospital work he wanted to take an early retirement and put into practice some of the more radical ideas that he had developed over the years. Pat and her husband, Canon Christopher Pilkington, had long been involved in healing and were enthusiastic about expanding their work. As for me, I was absolutely determined to do it. Keen wasn't the word, I was positively Messianic.

I was bursting with information about everything you could name. Our home was bristling with negative ionizers, orgone generators, water-filters, bean-sprouters, juicers, biofeedback machines and No Smoking signs and I was longing to share all this with other people. It had been the most awful struggle to find out what I wanted to know about all these things, to say nothing of the role of nutrition in cancer control, the use of vitamins and minerals, the value of healing, and I wanted to make it easier for others. Nobody should have to grapple with all this feeling as lost and alone as I had felt. There was the whole psychological side too. The cancer diagnosis brings you slap bang into a confrontation with your own mortality. Admittedly some people will duck this, save it for another day, but I couldn't believe I was the only person who had decided to try and deal with it now. My efforts to do so had been scrappy and erratic in the absence of good guidance and counselling. Cancer patients needed easy access to these services in addition to

76

physical therapy. Pat and I started mustering a team.

We met with all sorts of people: with counsellors, with psychologists, with healers, with organic gardeners, with people who ran health-food shops, yoga classes, medical centres. By the time Alec joined us for an all-day meeting at the Pilkingtons' home we already had a hard core of people who would help us.

We decided to give it a whirl. We would run a Centre as a pilot study and see what happened.

We started one day a week. We didn't advertise; if people needed us they would come.

They came.

That first week I sat in a circle of cancer patients and tried to explain how I had felt, what had happened to me. Within minutes two of them were weeping. I hesitated. Maybe I wasn't doing this right.

'Don't stop, please don't stop. I'm only crying because I'm relieved. I felt the same, but nobody listened.' 'I'm all right. I'm crying because I'm grateful to be allowed to feel this way.'

Everyone chimed in, sharing experiences that had only been cried into pillows, unlocking pain that had never been heard or healed. We had made a good beginning.

Time spent with Alec was unique for them all. Here was a doctor who explained things in a way that you could understand. He knew it was *your* cancer, not something happening in the hospital records, he gave you weapons to help you overcome it. He made himself available in a friendly, easy-going way, understood that you were afraid, let you have a cry if you wanted to.

Word spread around and people kept coming.

We were an entirely voluntary organization in those days. Nobody was paid and the patients came for nothing. We lived from hand to mouth, relying on occasional donations and the generosity of the Guy Pilkington foundation (a charitable trust for Christian ministry, healing and counselling) who kept a roof over our heads and the gas, water and electricity boards off our backs. Our telephone bill alone was like the national debt. Thousands of people owe the Guy Pilkington Foundation a great deal of gratitude. Without

77

their support we could not have existed then and would not exist now.

The Centre has been an unqualified success from the day we started, but we have always tottered along on a razor's edge financially. To begin with I was puzzled and annoyed that I couldn't raise the money we needed. Pat Seed had raised millions, why couldn't I? No doubt if I had been trying to raise money for a scanner I could have done the same. Something to support the existing establishment would have been easier to justify. The trouble with the Cancer Help Centre was that we were offering something the establishment didn't offer. It was very difficult not to look like an alternative or a threat.

By this time I had restarted my acupuncture practice. My own experience had deepened my understanding and this was reflected in my work. I was busier than ever. Gradually I started working longer and longer hours, squeezing my self-help therapies into an ever shortening lunchtime. In between seeing patients at home and fetching the children from school I was racing into Bristol for interminable meetings about the development of the Centre.

These meetings had to be seen to be believed.

In view of the fact that everyone involved in what we were doing tended to be the more receptive, feminine type of person, our discussions were never controlled by the natural boundaries of intolerance. As a result we all used to rabbit on, repeating ourselves, agreeing with each other, restating things until we were thoroughly exhausted and not necessarily a lot further forward. There was never any question of a majority decision, we all had to agree about everything. It was delightful really, but terribly inefficient. We had meetings that honestly lasted all day. We used to take packed lunches. By the end of these sessions we were all dizzy with tiredness. I remember Ludi Howe, a counsellor who joined us in the very early days, saying quite firmly at one such time, no thank you she did not want a glass of apple juice or a tisane of rose-hip, she wanted, 'a decent cup of lorry-driver tea!'

But we needed more than a short shot of tannin to put us on the right road.

It was obvious that the pilot study had been a success and the Centre was here to stay. We needed a more formal structure and set up a management committee which David agreed to chair. He managed to cut down the length of meetings by about half and attempted to organize us without bullying us. I can safely say without reference to him that it was the most trying job he has ever had, but he was the right person for it. One of my husband's most consistent, and as far as I'm concerned, most enviable, qualities, is that he doesn't mind what people think of him. Consequently he was tough enough to withstand all the complaints and disaffection that attend the unenviable task of creating order out of chaos, and survived the role of chairman for a year or so before handing this doubtful privilege over to Christopher Pilkington.

The patients kept coming, both to the Cancer Help Centre and to my practice at home. I was increasingly occupied with the role of therapist. I didn't really know if I was still a patient or not.

Cancer is such an invidious, idiosyncratic disease, and plays such sneaky tricks, it's hard for patients and doctors alike to be confident about the state of play at any given time. There are many examples of people being discharged with a 'clean sheet' from hospital, returning for check-ups a few months later only to be told they have secondaries. The cruel part of it all is that they may have been feeling perfectly well. So, the fact that I was feeling fine wasn't any kind of proof that I was not slowly building up a tumour somewhere else. It was very hard to know what to do. Did I have to carry on behaving like a patient in crisis for the rest of my life, or could I start tailing off the dramatic response a bit? It would be nice to soft pedal for a while, the whole family needed a break as well as me.

Somehow I never managed to serve lentils and vegeburgers in such a way as to give Heinz or McDonald's any cause for alarm. My children were coping as best they could, but their plaintive requests for 'proper food like everyone else has' when they had their friends to tea underlined for me how odd their lifestyle had become. It didn't seem fair to isolate them from their peer group in this way, but I suffered a positive torrent of emotions every time I pushed a few fish fingers round the frying pan. In my eyes they glowed with poisonous yellow colouring, and serving them up with chips, heavy with fatty floating-free radicals and cholesterol, made me feel like one of the Great English Poisoners, but what could I do? We needed a holiday.

To go cycling in France might have seemed an odd choice since we had never before cycled as a family – we didn't even own a bike each, but it was something I had always wanted to do. During times of despair and disappointment I had set myself goals, and one of them was to be well enough to take the children cycling in France. When such a goal seemed ludicrous I always had another, smaller goal, more easily achievable, to keep me going. When I was in Germany the small goal was to get home for Christmas, the crazy one was to learn to windsurf. I had seen my first sailboarder on the lake and he looked everything I wasn't – strong, powerful and in control – and for years I secretly nourished the longing to learn. I had been through such frightening and difficult times since getting home that occasionally the small goal was nothing more ambitious than getting through the day, but in the background lay the longing for cycling in France. It felt daring and adventurous and I was sick of being cautious and careful.

We did rustle up a decent bike each, but had no proper panniers, and the sight of our clothes bundled up in bags and strapped on the back was more reminiscent of a troupe of travelling tinkers than the tour de France. We were not well equipped. I dread to think what would have happened if it had rained.

Of course it didn't rain. The whole crazy trip was blessed from start to finish. We left at dawn, whispering with cloudy breath in the dew chilled air, through the sleeping village, along the cycle-track, past the curious, unmoving rabbits, arriving at Bath Spa station a good hour before the train. Jessica's fear that we would never actually get out of the country was reasonable enough for a ten year old who didn't even cycle to school. She had forced us all out of bed and on our way well in advance of necessity, but it seemed only reasonable to humour her. Her relief and sense of

80

achievement on merely reaching the station in time was a delight in itself.

As anyone who has taken a vehicle on a cross-Channel ferry will know, these boats are manned by chaps who have been hand-picked for their capacity to make you feel as silly and nervous as possible: whatever you do is wrong. It is just the same with a bike except for that fact that you run the additional risk of dying of carbon monoxide poisoning while you dart around from pillar to post trying to please the person who is shouting at you the loudest. We were too happy and excited and pleased with ourselves to care, wishing the journey away for the thrill of arriving.

David led our little troupe up the gang-plank and into St-Malo while I brought up the rear. (Essentially a role for an alert and agile member of the party since it required the fielding of all the odd socks and pairs of knickers that fought free of our bulging bags.) From this vantage point I was able to take a detached and objective view of David. His upper garments compensated in quantity for what they lacked in quality. He looked a bit bulgy. His paint-stained jeans were tucked into an awful pair of diamond-patterned cycling socks – the only bona fide piece of equipment we had between the lot of us. This vision was topped off with a woolly knitted hat that was sufficiently small for it to have risen up just a shade too far above his ears. He looked like Baden Powell in mufti. I wondered what on earth I looked like myself, the children certainly looked pretty funny. The French official waved us through, shaking his head in disbelief and brushing our passports to one side, murmuring, 'You are English of course.' As we wobbled on to French soil Jessica protested in wonder, 'How did he know we were English, Mummy?' and the holiday really began. How could we be anything else?

That night we all slept together in a room with two double beds and one single. We had to take it in turns to undress and pick our way between the tightly packed beds to the washbasin. We couldn't sleep for laughing. As soon as a minute of quiet had passed someone would snicker and set us all off again. We laughed until we cried, until bits of us that we didn't know existed started to ache. For five days we lived on top of each other, revelling in the closeness and intimacy. We were within sight and sound of each other all day, and sometimes all night. When we weren't all in the same room, there was much pyjama-clad scuttling between rooms and banging of messages on walls. We fell sideways into hedges with exhaustion going up hills, we were laughed at by athletes who flashed past us on racing bikes, we were greeted with delight and made a huge fuss of in all the little villages, we bought sumptuous picnics and lounged about in fields and on the beach and, best of all, we forgot all about cancer. It was the most glorious experience and we have repeated it since. For me it was the perfect antidote to all the separation and fear of the previous year.

Almost overnight the children seemed reassured that I was better. I was no more exhausted than they were. How could I be ill doing something as ordinary and silly as riding around on a bike. One night I was worried about finding something suitable for me on the menu and, asking the kitchen to prepare something specially for me, I saw Justine's face crumple with sadness. 'But I thought you were all right now ...'.

This was to become more and more of a problem. It is hard to maintain a lifestyle that is sensible and self-protective if it acts as a constant reminder to people that you are sick. Or have been sick. Or might be sick again. How do you lead a 'normal' life and not put yourself at risk? I was soon to learn that this was the $64 million question.

My breast seemed to have returned to normal. I felt happy and strong. I wanted someone to tell me I was cured. The trouble was, I didn't know who to ask. I didn't think my doctor would be impressed by my newly discovered ability to produce alpha-waves on a mind mirror, he was certainly unlikely to consider this as a sign of my recovery, much less as an acceptable alternative to a mastectomy. Also, I was shy of returning to the hospital I had left a year before. I toyed with the idea of contacting Issels, as he had asked me to do, but I had modified his instructions to the point where he would hardly have considered me to be using his therapy anyway. It had been difficult to get additional supplies of some of the homoeopathic injections and the enzyme preparations; I had stopped the fevers altogether after a few months. There hardly seemed any point in contacting him. I couldn't afford to go back to Germany anyway. We were still paying off debts from the last time.

Despite my enthusiasm about my excursions into different levels of consciousness, I wasn't sure whether what I was doing actually constituted a therapy or not. Of course I saw patients who came to Bristol making impressive improvements on the new diet, relaxation and vitamin routine, and this was wonderfully encouraging, but it was still true that all these people had undergone surgery, radiotherapy or chemotherapy before they came. It was painfully difficult to assess my own situation.

I decided to have homoeopathic treatment and rang a doctor who had been recommended to me. It would be so lovely to be seeing someone regularly, who might make some judgements about how I was getting on. I was still longing to have a healer other than myself.

'Oh yes,' she said, when I spoke to her on the telephone, 'I've heard about you.'

Good grief, what on earth had she heard? She didn't say. I explained that I was doing all sorts of things to help myself; a bit of Issels' therapy, a special diet, some vitamins and minerals, and of course having acupuncture treatment. She finally interrupted me.

'You'd have to stop all that if you want me to treat you. It's too confusing for me if my patients follow more than one therapy at once.'

'How can I do that? I understand that you can't offer me a cure, I feel I'd be mad not to do all I can to help myself ... I dare not put all my eggs in one basket ... I don't think I've got the courage to stop everything else.' I must have sounded as unhappy as I felt.

'I hope you don't feel I'm rejecting you or abandoning you or anything ...'

Yes, that was exactly how I felt.

What was the matter with all these people? This 'do it my way or I won't help at all' attitude. She was just the same as the doctors: locked up in a closed system that was more concerned with preserving its own integrity than risking exposure to imperfect patients. I was beginning to see that when you are ill and seeking help from someone else you are expected to perform in a certain way, preferably pretty passively but, if you must get involved and join in the healing process, then you must do what you are told. Surely there must be a compromise position between accepting help and being part of the decision-making process? Maybe, but I wasn't going to achieve it with this particular lady.

I held on to the belief that a relationship of mutual respect between therapist and patient must be possible, and I was soon to be rewarded. A few months later I met Dr Dorothy West and we embarked upon a voyage of discovery that has been a constant joy and source of excitement to us both. I started taking a day off work every few weeks and driving down to Plymouth to see her, usually staying for lunch and for as much of the afternoon as I dared, racing back along the motorway to meet my domestic commitments, singing all the way with the sheer pleasure at having found a twin soul. There was nothing about what I was doing or saying that she found at all odd. She thought my way of having cancer was wise and enlightened, but a tough course to follow, and she was going to help in every possible way. She gave me homoeopathic remedies, home-grown vegetables, hours and hours of her time and a renewed belief in myself. She is one of those rare beings who know how to work from the heart. She loved me. Just writing about her makes me feel good. She had the effect of making me feel powerful and effective. In simple terms, her treatment of me had an enabling effect. A useful characteristic for any doctor, but rare, very rare.

I talked so much about her David started coming too. One day he sneaked his way into her consulting room and I found myself outside waiting for him. They were an awfully long time in there. What was the matter with him that took so long to tell? Poor David! Trying to be my doctor, my analyst, my lover and my friend all rolled into one. Never knowing which role he would have to play next, always having to respond to my demands at the expense of his own needs, shielding me from my uncertainty by telling me all was well when he was far from certain that it was. Lonely as I felt at times, I always had him. Who did he have? Well, now he had

84

Dorothy. With her help we both moved more quickly and efficiently through the areas we wanted to explore, with a sense of relief that there was someone around who understood what we were trying to do. Dorothy showed great skill and subtlety in her handling of both of us. We have reason to be grateful to her.

David also occasionally joined in another of my regular routines. He often came with me to visit my healer.

This was an aspect of my cancer-care package that had started before I went to Germany.

During the chaotic and terrifying time that followed my leaving hospital and flying to the RingbergKlinik. Pat had suggested I should see a healer. Reared as I had been by the daughter of a Welsh preacher and the son of a Cornish Methodist, I took a dim view of things like healing. The fact that my attitude was based on ignorance in no way diminished its rigidity. In fact, quite the reverse: it was precisely because I didn't know anything about healing that enabled me to hold the view that it lay somewhere on a continuum between being a load of old nonsense and a form of black magic.

'No thanks Pat, I don't think it would help really.'

I was particularly prickly at this time. I had only just left hospital after the disastrous lump biopsy and was still at the stage of having to fend off my doctor's cynicism as well as my own. My suggestion that I might visit Issels, a fully-qualified medical practitioner who had been treating cancer for over thirty years, had met with explosive dismissal. I was keen not to get involved in anything else that might attract more negative attention.

'You'd love him, Pen, he's a marvellous person. Please let me bring him.'

'No, no, we're all right. I can't cope with that, don't bring him, please don't.'

She did.

David came from the telephone one afternoon.

'That was Pat, I'm afraid she's on her way with this healer bloke. You'll just have to put up with it, there's no stopping her.'

'Well you must sort them out. I can't handle this.'

I waited tensely, feeling irritable and anxious. What on earth would he do? Supposing he sank to his knees, or started waving his arms around ... supposing he started speaking in tongues ... I'd never forgive Pat for this. We heard the car draw into the drive and David looked through the window.

'Well, he can't be all bad, he's driving a bright red BMW.'

For some reason this struck me as being inordinately funny and as I laughed some of my fear subsided, and instead of darting away to my room as I had planned, I went out to meet him.

Another of the Gentle Giants.

For years now I have been going to see him. At least that's what I think I'm doing when I find my way to his exquisitely beautiful, freezing cold old rectory, buried in a walled, bird-song garden, in the depths of Somerset. I imagine I'm going to see him, but while I'm there it's God I feel close to, and really I think it's Him I'm going there to find.

From that first day, as the BMW engine cooled outside and he bounded upstairs to my room, he started a process in me that has continued ever since. I could tell you no more about healing now than I could before. I don't know what 'it' is, I don't know how 'it' works. I only know that Tim's prayerful, loving belief in my wholeness has been instrumental in my coming nearer to achieving it.

True to form, my first encounter with him was emotional and tearful. In between my sobs he asked, 'What do you most wish that healing could give you?'

A little voice inside me snapped back that I wanted not to have cancer, of course, not to have a leaky hole in my breast, not to be in pain, but I listened, stunned, to the sound of my own voice saying, 'Most of all I want proper judgement.'

I listened to myself saying this with some surprise, but I was right, and I would say the same thing now.

Perhaps that is one of the things that healers do, release within you a proper perception of your needs. I only know that, having dithered and worried endlessly about whether or not to go to Germany, by the following morning I was in no doubt. We were going, if only for a look around.

Since I spent such a long time in Germany I didn't see Tim again for months, but sometimes during my mountain walks in Bavaria I would find myself suddenly stopping in my tracks and standing quite still, knowing that he was praying for me. I could go back today and mark the exact spot where this first happened to me, it was so powerful and strange, but over the weeks I grew quite used to it.

Once I was back in England I started going to see him regularly. As with nearly everything else I was doing I wasn't quite sure why I was doing it. It is true that these healing sessions always and invariably helped the pain, but I was fortunate in that I did not have very much to cope with in that department, and this was never my motive for going. What I was seeking was more elusive than that. I always felt stronger and more confident when I came away, and pleasantly peaceful, but the overall feeling was that of having clicked into place. The nearest analogy I can come up with is to do with memories of tracing very complicated geography maps with lots of islands and wiggly coastlines and borders. When you line your tracing up with the original, if it is fractionally off-centre then the whole thing looks a chaotic jumble, but suddenly there is that satisfying moment when all the bits fit and the map is meaningful again. Every time I drove away from Tim I used to feel as though a detailed and complex tracing of my internal circuits and self had been adjusted to fit. I felt more in line with myself. Of course, it is hardly likely that any two people would have similar responses to healing, indeed most people might have rather different expectations of it in the first place.

Certainly I noticed at Bristol a wide variety of ways in which patients approached the idea of healing. Some saw it as a specifically religious thing, a way of drawing closer to God and feeling more at peace with themselves. Others were uncompromisingly material in their attitude to healing and their expectations were all focused on the physical plane. They were hoping for their tumours to shrink or their cancers to go away. I am in no doubt that healing can be breathtakingly effective in this sphere, but I am not sure that we can insist on it being so. I think that the looser and freer we are in our expectations then the more likely we are to get the healing we need, and that may not be what we think we need, or what we want.

It wasn't surprising that David should have presented himself for healing. After all, he had never played the role of passive observer of my self-discovery trip, he had eaten the diet, risked himself with Dorothy West, and generally tended to join in whenever possible. I couldn't say what benefits he felt accrued to him when he took the wing chair in Tim's study, but the fact that he did it more than once speaks for itself. I do know, however, that he always fell deeply asleep afterwards, relying on me to drive him home dead to the world.

One day my father-in-law asked me to take him as well.

He was deteriorating fast and was very ill. He had pinned his hopes firmly on the hospital and had done everything they suggested. His last dose of chemotherapy however had been such a terrible experience that he said he would prefer to die than go through that again. There was never any question that the treatment would cure him or bring about a significant remission. It was only a question of maybe controlling the cancer for a bit longer. He was going to die anyway. He found the treatment so unbearable he preferred sooner than later.

'Do you think they'll mind if I say I don't want any more treatment?'

'Mind! What do you mean, "mind", it's your body, it's your choice.' But I knew perfectly well what he was worried about, I had heard it so many times from others.

'Maybe if I don't do what they want, they won't look after me any more. You know, be there when I need them. You know what I mean.'

Isn't it incredible that the confusion of roles in medicine and healing should have led to this? Of course it is inconceivable that any doctor would withdraw support from a dying patient as a kind of revenge, a punishment for not doing as he was told, but the truth is that many patients do actually fear that this will happen, and they adapt and modify their behaviour towards their doctors as a result.

It is easy to see that doctors are staggering around under

the impossible burden that society's expectations has placed on them. We expect them to put everything right – which is an absurd expectation. They have been taught that they usually can – which is equally absurd. Consequently, when the scientific myth is blown and things start going wrong we, as patients, start throwing blame and accusations, we may even call in solicitors and sue. In response to this the doctor may do any one of a number of things, but he certainly isn't going to take this blame on board himself. And no more should he. However, he shouldn't try and bounce it back to the patient either.

This is a problem for any therapist in any field. What do we do when things start going wrong? If, despite our best efforts, the patient gets worse? When what we tell them to do, or do to them, doesn't make them better? What guilty little hook inside of us latches on to the fear and pain that such a situation creates? Why does somebody have to be blamed for it?

Looking for somebody to blame is only a weak response to a challenging situation, but by falling into it we are expecting other people to feel guilt and perhaps even shame. This may make us feel a bit better for a while, but the terrible trilogy of guilt, blame and shame are best avoided altogether.

Daddy didn't want any more treatment and finally plucked up the courage to say so. He didn't want any advice from me either. He was delighted to see me looking so well on what was now affectionately referred to as my jungle juice and mental gymnastics, but it didn't appeal to him. If he couldn't have smoked salmon sandwiches then life wasn't worth living anyway. He knew himself better than most.

He came down to stay.

'How are you doing then? What are they saying at the hospital?'

'Don't buy any long playing records, or get engrossed in any TV serials. Something like that.'

He really meant us to laugh, and we did. He was still the best company for miles around right up until he died.

I was surprised when he asked to see Tim, and I never knew what he expected to get out of it, but a healing took place that certainly surprised me. Waiting for him to finish his session I wandered into the Norman church that all but sits on Tim's front lawn. Shivering on a scratchy pew I knew for the first time that my father-in-law loved me. That he had forgiven me.

It had been so hard for him, my not being Jewish. Everything was made worse by the fact that he liked me so much, we enjoyed each other's company, made each other laugh. But I lacked the one essential characteristic that he was looking for, and for years this had lain as an unbridged barrier between us.

When my son Daniel was born we had him circumcized. This had been difficult to arrange because of our so-called 'mixed' marriage, but eventually pressure from the Jewish side of the family persuaded the *mohl* to come to the house to do the honours. Things didn't go very well. Daniel bled a lot and there was a buzz of panic and prayers. I was terrified. Wisely my mother-in-law took over and I fled to my room, cursing myself for ever subjecting my most precious, beloved infant to such a torture. Daddy found me hugging myself by the window trying not to scream out my fear and panic. He knew that this circumcision was my sacrifice for him, that I wanted it to please him.

'This doesn't make him Jewish you know.'

I didn't think it would, but I'd hoped it might help. Of course it wasn't enough, nothing would ever be enough. Over the years we grew closer and closer, but there was always that little corner of reservation. I gave up dreaming that one day he would be glad that his son had married me. Me, not some nice suitable little Jewish girl, but me. He was generous, affectionate and full of praise for me, but I always felt I had let him down.

It was very strange to be taking him to a healer – a retired priest furthermore – and, while waiting for him, frozen to my seat, to be overwhelmed by the knowledge that the last barrier was down. I don't pretend to understand why this unconditional love could only be released through suffering, but it was so.

We drove home talking of inconsequential nothings and for the last few months of his life we were inseparable. It was a relationship worth waiting fifteen years for.

Months later, on impulse, I took the train up to see him. Astonishment vied with delight.

'What have you come for?'

'I've come for tea.'

'No, no, seriously, what have you come for?'

'Nothing else. I've come to see you.'

He held me and cried a little and tried to say what he felt, and couldn't. I said I knew what he felt, so no need to say it.

'I don't believe in anything afterwards, you know. Not like you do.'

'I don't think that matters. I believe it for you, that's enough. You just come and meet me when it's my turn, I'll see you there.' And I will, I will. At the Judah gate.

We drank tea and I went home. Over two hundred miles for a cup of tea and a taste of immortality. One of the best days I've ever had.

It may seem a bit excessive that two people should have to have life-threatening diseases before they finally get their act together, but the healing of this relationship brought a peace to my life that made it all the sweeter. And, strange as it may seem, my uncertainty about my future survival was more bearable as a result. It was another bit of unfinished business that had finally been resolved and could come off the agenda.

Chapter 6

Keep your mouth shut
Guard the senses
And life is ever full.
Open your mouth
Always be busy
And life is beyond hope.
                              Lao Tsu

Within a year of coming back from Germany I was feeling full of strength and optimism. My breast felt fine, the rest of me seemed in good shape and I was having a great life.

It was just as well I was feeling better, I needed all the energy I could muster to maintain a lifestyle of ever-increasing pressure.

Despite a conscious attempt on our part to keep a low profile, demand for the Cancer Help Centre was growing all the time. We had a ludicrously long waiting list that caused people to burst into tears of despair on the telephone when hearing how long it would be before they would be able to come. We were for ever squeezing in 'just one more' with the result that some people had to eat their lunch standing up, there was a permanent queue for the lavatory and endless complaints from our neighbours about the parking.

We increased our commitment from one day a week to two, then from two to three. The pressure on our volunteer force was very great and eventually we had to start paying some of our therapists and, most reluctantly, making a token charge to the patients. It was obvious that the need was for a full-time Centre with properly paid personel, but that was an enormous step, and we simply did not have the money necessary to take it. In order to run the Centre we had it was essential that some people continued to work for nothing. Fortunately there have always been enough of us who do to keep our noses just above the water.

We were all working longer and harder hours. Because of this I was trying to force my acupuncture practice to fit into what time I had left and started work earlier each day. I used to dive into my white coat as the children left for school in the mornings and struggle out of it as they came home in the afternoons. Then I started cooking the supper and helping with homework. If my 12.30 client was late and my 2 o'clock client early then I didn't get a lunch-hour worthy of the name.

I had never been so much in demand or so successful. I was dashing in and out of Bristol, attending conferences, giving talks, reading articles about myself in magazines, watching myself on television and helping to make a series of programmes for BBC2 about the Cancer Help Centre.

I was spending a lot of time grappling with things of great pith and moment, and less and less time on either being myself or looking after myself. Little things like trudging around the supermarket with a trolley were a real treat.

Naturally everyone else could see the danger of this, but I couldn't be told. Well, I could be told, but I didn't listen. Even that's not true, I listened. I just didn't take any notice, I knew better. I believed that because I had shouted 'bugger' to the mountains and said 'no' to a few unreasonable requests that I now knew all about identifying and protecting myself; about being myself and not what other people wanted me to be. Since the issue had been revealed to me and I had acknowledged it I believed that I had dealt with it once and for all.

I had yet to learn that freeing oneself from the sticky grip of the politics of the protestant ethic, with its attractive rewards for deeds and performance, is like wrestling with an octopus. If one tentacle doesn't get you, another one will.

I was zapping around like Wonder Woman with stars on my shorts, doing good deeds and loving every minute.

In my eyes this was different from the frantic overworked

performance I had indulged in before I was ill. I had been like it because I had felt I had to justify my existence by being useful. Because I didn't feel so small about myself now I couldn't believe I was making the same mistake again. I was flashing about keeping up this punishing schedule now because what I was doing was 'right'. I was 'making a positive contribution to the world', any minute now I would turn into a 'terribly nice person'. My rewards for over-working in the past had been to feel I had a right to exist, this time they were much juicier. I was getting an enormous amount of encouragement in the form of affection, praise and approval.

Anyway, if I was going to modify my performance at all that meant I had to say 'no' to somebody who needed me. Never my strong suit.

Only Tim managed to penetrate my armour of self-justification. He tried to tell me it wasn't my job to save the world single-handed without a tea-break.

'Remember, it's much easier to do than to be.'

And how.

Of course what I was doing was important, but it was distracting me from finding my still point. I had passed from being so receptive and impressionable I was practically falling over backwards, to being so thrusting and dynamic I was buzzing around like a clockwork toy. I was still a long way from being single-weighted. Perhaps you have to experience both extremes before you can balance in the middle. I know I had to.

At around this time I decided to tackle another of my 'impossible' goals. Ever since my first sight of the windsurfer on Lake Tegernsee I had secretly harboured the idea that one day I would be the strong, powerful person kicking up the bow-wave, not the awed little weakling that looked on admiringly. We took a family holiday in a rather tatty flat in Spain, where, as I had hoped, the beach boasted a modest sailboard school. In an attempt to spare myself a good deal of teasing and advance humiliation, I decided to sneak off secretly in the morning at a ridiculously early hour and make my first try without even telling my family. My plan was to have daily lessons and then make my first appearance before

94

them skimming elegantly across the bay, greeting their astonished cries of admiration with an airy wave of the hand.

This fantasy was rapidly dispersed due to the fact that on day two I couldn't lift my arms above shoulder level. I seemed quite normal in every other respect. I could even clean my teeth unaided, but brushing my hair was out of the question. It is difficult in any circumstances to ask your husband to start doing your hair for you without offering some kind of explanation, but especially fraught for us since we were still vulnerable to the idea that every physical change that took place in me might be a 'sinister sign'. It didn't seem fair to leave anyone wondering if this was a symptom of advanced bone secondaries, even though my explanation for my painful semi-paralysis was met with a lot of ribald mockery.

'Are you telling me that half-an-hour of pulling wet sails out of the water can do this to you? I should quit now while you can.'

Now fully wised up to my plot, everyone insisted on pushing in, the men in particular, smugly confident that this would not be a hard act to beat. But there is some justice in the universe. Daniel gave up almost immediately, never quite sure if he was going backwards or forwards, and not prepared to continue making a fool of himself long enough to find out. David was more persistent. Clearly he too harboured visions of himself spinning off over the horizon on one toe, and he was puzzled at his apparent inability to achieve this within the space of a few minutes. I cannot deny that his total ineptitude made my modest, but undeniably superior, performance all the sweeter. After a few days of imagining that changing the board, changing the sail and even waiting for the wind to change would improve his dexterity he was finally and ignominiously rescued from the rocks and the jelly fish by a man in a pedalo. This humiliation was exacerbated by the fact that his rescuer, having safely installed David on his humble craft, then proceeded to sail the surf-board round and round him shouting explanations and instructions throughout the return journey. This unrewarding experience had the dual effect of convincing David never to set foot on a board ever again, and set him in unreasonable awe of my own achievements. Naturally I lapped this up and showed off like mad.

In time I could sail a full circuit of the bay and comb my hair all by myself the following morning. I had laid another ghostly image of myself as a helpless, sick victim. Of course this messing about on the board had a much deeper significance for me than the average holidaymaker. One afternoon the weather changed, the wind blew up quite spitefully and it turned cloudy and cold. By the time I finally staggered up the beach I found, to my surprise, that it was empty of all but the man who ran the surf school. He sat huddled against the elements under his kagoul and greeted me in his soft, Dutch voice:

'I knew you would be English, the English never give up. You fight with this board as if your whole life depended on it.'

In a funny kind of way I think it did.

Within two years of being a wreck in a lay-by I was back on the track again, within four years I was tearing along in the fast lane. Perhaps I might have made the necessary adjustments to my now somewhat frenetic lifestyle without having to come to grief first, but something happened that I found extremely difficult to handle.

When I talked to Dorothy about the BBC '40 minutes' programmes she had warned me, 'You're dealing with very powerful forces there, you must be very careful.'

I was soon to understand what she meant.

The television team were lovely. They came to make one programme and stayed to make six. They were sensitive, thoughtful and caring. They didn't give anyone a hard time, they didn't intrude. They formed close, personal relationships with both patients and therapists and we liked them. Nevertheless Dorothy was right, we were tinkering with powerful forces.

For weeks at a time we sweated under bright lights and tripped over trailing wires. The crew contributed their own energy to the place, making tea, offering lifts, alerting us to patients' needs as they saw them. An unusual and moving experience for us all. They tried to understand us, and – even more important – they tried to project that understanding accurately in the programmes. By and large they did that very well, but I was in for a shock.

We were all interviewed quite a bit and miles and miles of film was taken with the patients. We didn't know quite what to expect when we sat down to watch the rushes of the first programme, but I had a vague idea it would be a sort of composite picture of what we were doing. Instead of this I watched myself, or a part of myself, monopolizing a good three-quarters of the first programme. The second was almost as bad.

Watching oneself on television is the most unnerving experience. I could see that the person up there waving her arms around and telling them how it is, that that person was me, but it wasn't the whole of me. How could it be? The media only ever deals in cameos, or fragments, and there is a great deal of selecting and rejecting that goes on. I was being presented, sensitively and kindly presented, as a clever, strong, perceptive person, with an answer to everything. Like I said, Wonder Woman, with stars on her shorts.

No doubt the nervous wreck that cried all the time was curling up on the cutting room floor.

I was not smart enough to laugh at this. Somewhere inside me there was a part of myself that took it seriously. I picked up this image and tried to maintain it. I felt increasingly that I had to stay well, be fit and healthy, radiate happiness and contentment, and generally keep up with what was now a bright, shiny glittering persona. Overnight I changed from being an uncertainty to being a success.

One of my friends, suffering from Hodgkin's disease, said, 'If anything happened to you Penny, we'd all give up.' Something had gone horribly wrong somewhere.

Meanwhile all sorts of exciting things were happening. The television programmes had precipitated an avalanche of interest in the Centre. Our mail was being delivered by the sack-load, the telephone was jammed night and day. Not only patients, but doctors and nurses and all sorts of therapists were desperate to get in touch. They too wanted to expand their understanding of how to handle the cancer crisis. More accurately, they wanted to learn how to handle any crisis.

The least expected and most touching aspect of the sudden burst of publicity was that it triggered off a response from people who have never had cancer or anything to do with it. For months afterwards I was stopped in the shops, on the streets, once in the Pump Rooms at Bath, by such people.

'Listening to you took me back to how I felt when my son was killed.'

'I'm sure you're right dear, we all need to deal with our problems that way.'

'Do you have to have cancer to come to your Centre? I really want to come, but I'm afraid I don't think I've got it.' This was another one who, any minute now, was going to tell me how lucky I was to have had it.

Perhaps the funniest incident of all took place on a cross-Channel ferry. We had the doubtful privilege of being aboard the only boat to risk istelf in a force 9 gale, with some quite interesting results. There must have been other passengers aboard beside myself and the children, who were not sick, but it was hard to believe it. Apart from the misery of so much human suffering the stewards were kept busy by the damage to the fittings of the boat itself. Every few minutes there was a terrible crash and the sound of broken glass. The Space Invaders machines were flung about and reduced to rubble; the duty free shop was awash with liquor; and regular tannoy announcements requested that the owners of certain vehicles should present themselves at the Purser's office, please. Presumably to take away what was left of their cars in a couple of carrier bags. Pandemonium was the word. David had gone away to die under the stairs where he lay shivering and sweating, and it was while I was on my way to see if I could do anything for him that the boat suddenly dropped away from under my feet. At least, that's how it seemed. To the accompaniment of a cacophany of shrieks and bangs, I was knocked off my feet and thrown across what was left of the lounge, I ended up in a painful heap, mercifully within grasp of a handrail, and hauled myself up, nose to nose with a young girl as bruised and dishevelled as I was. Her eyes widened in recognition.

'You're the lady on the television programmes!' It was all I could do to stop her discussing the meaning of life then and there.

As the weeks and months went by it became increasingly obvious that the programmes had touched off a response common to everyone who watched them, not just the cancer sufferers. I found myself inundated with requests for acupuncture. If people couldn't qualify for admission to the Centre by having cancer they could manage the odd rheumaticky knee, the occasional headache or two. They came ostensibly for treatment, but most of them were seeking a much more profound healing. Holistic therapists are accustomed to many a tear being shed in their rooms, but the sort of pain and need that started to pour out in mine was of an altogether different order.

During this time I was deeply influenced by my relationship with Ainslie Meares. I had first come across him in Germany where I read a book he had written entitled *Cancer, Another Way*. To say that I read it is not quite correct: I devoured it. It fell apart with so much handling and I carried it around wrapped in a rubber band. I could recite whole pages of it by heart. Of course I could, I had written it myself. Well, I might just as well have done, it was such a perfect expression of what I was thinking. I dreamed of going to see him, but this was an absurd fantasy since I couldn't really afford to be in Germany, never mind the other side of the world.

To my delight he cropped up again in my life during the bio-feedback sessions with Maxwell Cade, who frequently quoted from Ainslie's work. It was inevitable that I should meet him, and since I couldn't get to him, he was brought to me.

One day when I was visiting Tim he mentioned that Australian friends of his had recommended an acquaintance of theirs to visit the rectory and talk about his work. I knew at once it would be him.

'That's Ainslie Meares isn't it?'

'Good heavens, how did you know that?'

It was certainly no surprise that my meeting with him should have been so wonderful, but I was delighted that he felt the same. In reply to my question as to why he had come to Europe – assuming a conference or family visit – he smiled and said softly, 'To meet you of course.'

From my point of view he was an answer to prayer: a doctor who thought that cancer was inextricably linked with unresolved conflicts and anxieties. Not only that, he believed that only the profound and prolonged reduction of stress would bring about its control or reversal. He had treated hundreds of patients who had benefited greatly from the atavistic meditation he taught, but they had all come to him at the end of the high technology trail. He was beginning to despair of ever meeting anyone who wanted to deal with disease in this way from day one. If your friends are your needs answered, then we were destined to be very close.

During an exchange of letters he wrote:

'There are two kinds of anxiety, situational and existential. Anxiety from unconscious conflicts is still situational. Existential anxiety is the anxiety of being alive.'

What better than cancer, the threat of death, to trigger off such anxiety? Small wonder the Centre was attracting people who, to all intents and purposes were 'cured' of their cancer, but who were still raw with the pain of much deeper suffering. No surprise either that people dimly aware of their needs on this level felt having cancer would be a small price to pay for the chance to heal themselves. We had sounded a note that brought an avalanche cascading down around us.

Even Wonder Woman was struggling a bit.

At the Centre we decided that the need for much larger premises of our own, which we could run full-time, was now so great we would have to do something soon. We borrowed an enormous amount of money and bought Grove House, confident that we would be able to pay it all back and be self-financing before long. We haven't managed it yet, but we're on our way.

Almost as confirmation that we had done the right thing, Prince Charles came down and opened the new building for us.

He is a powerful and impressive man, and whatever difficulties he may or may not be having with the role of

100

service placed on him, it was exciting and encouraging to know that our future king has such an enlightened and sophisticated understanding of the need for healing. How appropriate and fortunate that the intuitive longing of so many ordinary people should be so well understood, indeed shared, by the family at the head of their state. It was a wonderful day.

Driving home through the blazing July heat, we reflected on the events of the last few years. Was it really only four years ago that I had walked out of hospital, seeking something that simply didn't exist? Had we managed to create something to fill for others the terrible void that had surrounded me then? We had, we really had. Maybe I could ease back a bit now.

I could and did, but the damage had been done. I had another lump in the same breast.

Chapter 7

Heal life if you can, with respect – but do not tamper wastefully with disease within a person's destiny. The ostensible result of such cures will be living corpses, individuals who no longer have access to spiritual power because they have bought off a serious disease with their souls.

Richard Grossinger

For several months I had been aware that changes were taking place in my breast. It didn't feel as soft as the other one and the nipple was being dragged slightly inwards. For some time there had been a suspicion of another lump, very close to the site of the last one, and so bound up with the old scar tissue it was difficult to identify for sure. Unfortunately it was defining itself more clearly every day and something else, most peculiar, was happening. Quite independent of the new lump was a wide patch of breast that had started thickening.

I consulted various doctors – hand-picked not to give me a hard time – and they all said the same thing.

'The thick patch is just a resolution of the haematoma you had from the lump biopsy – nothing to worry about at all. I don't know what to make of this other thing. Better have it looked at.'

I started looking after myself a bit better and hunted around for someone to tell me what I wanted to hear – that everything was all right. As if I would have believed it if I had heard it.

Then Ernesto came. Ernesto Contreras, dreadful irritant to the American FDA, running a cancer clinic just over the border in Mexico where people could get Amygdalin (variously known as laetrile or B17), good advice, tender loving care, and all sorts of other harmless and helpful anti-cancer agents. The ultimate holistic practitioner, he has a hospital too where patients can undergo surgery, radio-therapy or chemotherapy if appropriate. He was on a lecture tour and agreed to come to the Centre and talk to our own and any other interested doctors.

He and his wife stayed the night with Pat, and David and I entertained them the following day. We took them to Bath. They dutifully trailed around the Georgian terraces and enthused over the mysteries of the Roman Baths. We joined the multi-racial army of sightseers that was fighting its way round the city and dragged them from one attraction to another – little knowing that they would one day have their revenge.

When they had seen so much they could not politely take in anything else, we felt we could retire with honour from the tourist scene, and they did some shopping. I must confess that searching out cashmere sweaters in the heat of a spectacularly good summer had its funny little moments, and I did wonder in passing what possible use such garments would be in sunny Mexico, but it was a delightful day. We were all absolutely exhausted, of course, and collapsed at home for an hour of rest and recuperation before setting out for the evening lecture at the centre.

Ernesto had seen the television programmes.

'You are a real star! Wonderful, really wonderful.'

I thought he would be a good person to talk to about the not-so-wonderful parts.

He examined my breast. He asked me questions I couldn't answer about the results of the biopsy done four years before. Was it a hormone-dependent tumour for a start? I didn't know, how on earth would *I* know? Josef Issels, a fully qualified doctor with goodness knows how many years of experience hadn't managed to wrestle a copy of the laboratory report out of anyone, although he had tried hard enough, what chance did I have?

'This would be useful to know. What you are doing to save yourself is wonderful, but if every month you supply hormones that encourage cancer cells to grow, then this is very grave. Maybe you cannot keep ahead of this, perhaps this is why you have another lump.'

'What do you think I should do?'

'You must know this about the hormones. I think you should have this lump examined. The other thick part is nothing. Do not worry about that.'

Everyone seemed agreed on that at least, so I cheered up a bit.

'But you should do this quickly. This is urgent.'

Oh my God, here we go again.

His talk that evening at the Centre was a terrific success.

I have deliberately delayed describing what Ernesto is like because it is so difficult to do so without making him sound like a cross between an avenging angel and Luke the beloved physician. But by the end of his talk I wasn't the only one who would have described him thus and he was given the accolade he deserved. Nothing I could ever write about him could describe the sort of man he is better than the leaflet that he distributed to everyone there that night.

1 Corinthians 13
Paraphrased for the physicians by Dr Ernesto Contreras, Sr.

1. Though I became a famous scientist or practising physician, and I display in my office many diplomas and degrees, and I am considered as an excellent teacher or convincing speaker, but have no LOVE, I am just a sounding brass or a tinkling cymbal.
2. And though I have the gift of being an unusual clinician making the most difficult diagnoses; and understand all the mysteries of the human body; and feel sure I can treat any kind of diseases, even cancer; but have no LOVE, I am nobody.
3. And though I invest all my money to build the best facilities, buy the best equipment, have the most prominent physicians for the sake of my patients; and I devote all my time for their care, even to the point of neglecting my own family or myself; but have not LOVE, it profiteth me nothing.
4. LOVE is an excellent medicine, it is non-toxic; it does not depress the body defense, but enhances it.
5. It can be combined with all kinds of remedies, acting as a wonderful positive catalyst.
6. It relieves pain and maintains quality of life at its best level.
7. It is tolerated by anyone; never causes allergies or intolerance.
8. Common medicines come and go. What was considered good

yesterday, is useless now. What is considered good now will be worthless tomorrow. But LOVE has passed all tests and will be effective always.

9. We now know things only partially, and most therapies are only experimental.

10. But when all things are understood we will recognise the value of love.

11. It is the only agent capable of creating good rapport between patients, relatives and doctors, so everybody will not act as children but as mature people.

12. Today many truths appear as blurred images to us as physicians and we can't understand how the things of the spirit work to maintain life; but one day we will see all things very clearly.

13. And now remain three basic medications: Faith, Hope and Love, but the greatest of these is LOVE.

If this remarkable man is beginning to sound too good to be true I should add that one of his most endearing qualities is that he doesn't take himself too seriously. Whatever he does is always punctuated with laughter and good humour.

I considered myself fortunate to have been able to consult him and decided to take his advice. I felt it would be better for everyone if I didn't enter the ring for round two with my local hospital and decided to consult an oncologist a nice, safe hundred miles away.

He was very puzzled. Like everyone else he dismissed the large mass, which by this time was pulling my breast out of shape and causing the nipple to indurate, as being the side effect of so much internal bleeding years before. It was the other lump that confused him.

'If I had to guess, or make a judgement without any other evidence I would say that was a harmless fibro-adenoma. Obviously I can't be certain of that without taking tissue samples, but that's what I would expect to find.'

I was delighted, but surprised. 'I imagined you would think it must be sinister – with my history and so on.'

He looked a bit uncomfortable at this and said, 'Well I must admit I'm wondering if you ever had cancer in the first place.'

'What are you saying! For what other possible reason would they have wanted to do a mastectomy straight away?

They were full of all sorts of grim tales of what would happen to me if I didn't have further surgery and not promising much of a future if I did. It must have been cancer. Nobody would have made that sort of song and dance about anything else.'

'Yes, yes, that's true, but it's a bit difficult to square that with the present position. That was four years ago and here you are looking a picture of health having had an untreated cancer for all that time.'

Untreated!

I sat there, awash with oxygenated, lightly boiled blood, rattling with homoeopathic remedies, brimful of vitamins and minerals, aglow with negative ions, the faithful infuser of who knows what herbal fixes, able to produce alpha-waves at the drop of a hat, having re-cycled more organically grown food than a small market-garden, only to hear that I hadn't had any treatment.

'I don't suppose you see it quite that way,' he added hastily, 'but, from my point of view you've been untreated.'

The logic seemed to go something like this: either you didn't have cancer before and it isn't cancer now, or you do have cancer now, but you still didn't have it before because if you did you would not be here.

No doubt the results of this particular investigation were going to be as interesting to him as they were to me. Naturally he chased the information he wanted about my past history more successfully than Josef Issels had managed to do, and agreed that I had indeed had cancer four years before. I was 'an interesting case'.

This must have been written in letters a foot high all over my notes because I attracted a peculiar kind of attention in hospital.

My consultant's right-hand man appeared with a posse of white-coated henchmen jossling keenly for a place around the bed, struggling to stay the right side of the curtain.

'This is a very interesting case,' he intoned. I was pleased to be 'a very interesting case' because it sounded a bit more acceptable than being 'a very threatening patient'. Perhaps I was making progress after all. Then, turning towards them with a meaningful look, he added, 'the one I told you about.'

I would have given a lot to have heard that little talk. Whatever he had said had made such an impression on one of the scuffling little team of camp followers that he took to visiting me when he came off duty, in a sincere and desperate attempt to understand what I was trying to say. One evening he came back and asked:

'What exactly do you mean when you say your "model of disease" is different from mine?' I had to laugh. Can you imagine anybody talking like that? I used to do it all the time. Mind you it's probably no bad encounter for a budding young doctor. I did at least credit him with having a model of disease in the first place, although I doubt if he had ever given a thought to any such thing.

It wasn't easy trying to explain my attitudes and feelings to anybody else at a time when I was going through a painful period of reassessment myself. Despite all my protestations that I wanted to be a healthier person, not a tumour-free body, I knew that I had hoped the two would go hand in hand. Perhaps I wouldn't have to face this dilemma again. Maybe it would be an innocent fibro-adenoma.

It wasn't.

Unlike love, cancer is not lovelier the second time around. It isn't any easier either.

I was shattered.

I'd given all I'd got and it wasn't enough. What more did I have to do for goodness' sake? I felt like Alice in Wonderland trying to negotiate her way into the garden, struggling with doors and keyholes and keys, agonising over 'drink me' bottles and 'eat me' buns. She was either too big or too small or the key was in the wrong place. My life had the look of a similar farce, everything was being deliberately obtuse and difficult. I had done my best. If that wasn't enough, what was? I was going to have to find out pretty soon because the atmosphere in the hospital was hotting up.

My consultant called me into his room for a talk. I thanked him for doing such a nice job on my breast. There wasn't a lot left of it now that people kept taking little bits of it away, but it was obvious that he had handled me carefully, there was hardly any bruising and it all looked very neat and tidy. As if fearing that I might have ideas about having a mastectomy he said very sadly, 'I'm afraid there's no question of further surgery, it's too widely infiltrated in the breast. You see, that other odd thickness is malignant too.'

That was a terrible blow. Fighting back the old, familiar tears I listened to his advice:

'Radiotherapy. I'll put you on to a colleague of mine. I'm sorry Mrs Brohn, I really am, but there's no point in you seeing me again, there's nothing more that I can do for you.'

Would I have let him do it if there was? I doubt it. I had no intention of seeing the radiotherapist either.

I was back in my familiar role of nursing a painful wound and a lot of doubts while trying to defend myself from well-meaning pressure. I decided to avoid most of the battles by simply not telling many people what had happened. Naturally my sisters came, bless them – literally hundreds of miles – clutching wilting flowers from gardens and Devon lanes, bringing unbearably poignant memories of carefree pasts and fierce, passionate reassurances of the future. It felt good to be in the arms of a sister – the youngest of the three of us – who had once staggered up the road outside our home wielding a sweeping brush twice as long as she was to ward off attack from the local hoodlums who had put her precious sisters to flight. I knew she would do the same for my cancer if she could.

One thing was said that lingered:

'Don't try and do this on your own strength, Pen. Give it to God.'

I wasn't too sure about that. I was in a ward full of people who prayed to God that the surgeons wouldn't find cancer only to wake up, breast removed, to the news that they had. I had done much the same myself. I knew God was intimately involved in all this, but I still wasn't sure where or how. I believed that God helped those who helped themselves and the trick was to find out what it was you had to do. What's more, I had been busy telling other people what to do. That was all very well coming from Wonder Woman, the big it-can-be-done success story, but would it have quite the same clout from a hospital bed?

I felt all the things you might expect: frightened, uncertain, guilty, confused, embarrassed, angry. But looking around the ward at other women in similar physical shape I knew that I had made some progress over the four years. I saw them buying the comfort they needed with their compliance. In return for being passive patients they were treated to warm, encouraging little encounters during the day from various members of their hospital team, and they were visibly inspired and cheered by this. Gradually all the black panic that had engulfed them on hearing their diagnosis was being soothed away and forgotten. I knew, even more certainly than I had known before, that this was not right for me. I had to operate on the darkness that the experience exposed, not the experience itself. Unfortunately this meant I didn't qualify for the same comforting little chats – how could I? They didn't have anything to talk to me about if I wasn't going to have any more treatment.

As before, I had to ask myself why I couldn't do both: get my emotional and physical act together at the same time. The answer was still the same: I didn't trust myself. My hold on my inner development was better than it had been, but it was still very fragile. I couldn't risk the distraction or the redeployment of energy that would result if I started concentrating on a material path. Of course there was a sense in which I was already putting an enormous amount of energy into physical, material methods. The metabolic therapy, the vitamins and minerals, even the diet were all on the verges of the same path, but I knew from my experience of these approaches that they led me onwards all the time towards understanding myself as a whole. These methods required me to play an active role in my recovery, forced me to move from being a passive recipient of other people's methodologies towards being an active participant in my own healing process. In this way I could wriggle out of the feelings of fatalism and helplessness that accompanied the role of recipient, and start developing feelings of responsibility which made me feel more potent. But it was still true that I felt instinctively slightly antagonistic to the standard cancer therapies. They all seemed so gross and crude and unsubtle. I felt that blundering around with such massive weapons was not my style.

I was sure there was a way through this maze, and just

109

because I hadn't found it at the first turning didn't mean I would never find it. There was no reason for not continuing to try. Even if I never sorted it out properly, people learn from the failure of others just as certainly as by their success.

Back to the drawing board.

I mused over what the present situation indicated about my years of do-it-yourself cancer cures. Had they been a total failure, a partial success or a total success? It seemed to depend on who you asked. The surgeon had been surprised that I could have survived at all with my so-called 'untreated' tumour, so presumably, in his eyes I had been pretty clever. However, I had already had more than a hint from unsympathetic sources, ('I knew you should have had the mastectomy') that suggested there were others who thought I had been wasting my time.

Of course I had to face the fact that I had become pretty casual about my therapies over the last two years. I was not now nearly as fussy about diet and took a fairly haphazard vitamin and mineral dose – as much because I vaguely feared I might overdose in the long term as for any reason of neglect. Reluctantly I had to admit that hours of meditating and relaxing had been whittled down to a few minutes snatched here and there. But surely my life couldn't be hanging in a balance so sensitive that it tipped you into the grave if you substituted rose-hip with a few cups of Earl Grey tea every now and again? Of course it was just possible that I had cut too many corners and that a return to the old regime was all that I needed, but I was a bit wary of just doing more of the same. That smacked somewhat of the 'try harder' syndrome, a belief system most precious to the average school teacher but not to me. I have a drawer full of old school reports that insisted. 'She could do better if she tried harder.'

I didn't believe that then and I wasn't any more attracted to the idea now. I had tried as hard as I could. I had done all that I was capable of and achieved all that I was able to achieve. It seemed naïve to imagine that I actually could try any harder or that such an effort would result in a different outcome. I felt that a bit of lateral thinking would be more profitable.

My head was buzzing with all the things I had done in the

110

past and all the other things I'd heard of but hadn't done. No doubt they were all pieces of an enormous jigsaw that only required being put together in the correct way to produce a nice clear picture.

I felt a bit like Eric Morecombe who, producing the most appalling cacophany of sound when purporting to play the piano with André Previn, replied to Previn's exasperated insistence that he wasn't playing the right notes, by saying, 'I am playing the right notes, but not necessarily in the right order.'

No doubt the solution to my problem was all in there somewhere, but I was beginning to wonder if it would take me as long to sort it out as it would take the proverbial six monkeys to type the entire works of Shakespeare.

Not a happy time.

I was very well treated during my week in hospital. The staff were puzzled but always kind. I decided to ask one of them to tell the radiotherapist not to come. It seemed such an awful waste of his time, and I dreaded having to go through the whole tearful trauma of trying to explain myself. I had done this so many times one might have expected me to make a reasonably good job of it by now, but, far from becoming easier, I was more garrulous and incoherent with each attempt. I was becoming more inarticulate and muddled every time I opened my mouth, and if that's how it sounded to me I could only imagine how it sounded to somebody else. I decided it was better to let the radiotherapy department think I was plain scared, I was too exhaused for anything else. I would tell sister to put the radiotherapist off or, if he insisted on speaking to someone, he could see David.

Before I could put this plan into action, he arrived. I had lost control of the situation before we even began and I didn't know what to do. Fortunately he elected to bat first.

Dr Howard sat down on the end of the bed. Now that was nice for a start, at least I didn't have to gaze up at him reverentially, but could make eye contact on the level. Did I want the curtains closed around us or not? You mean that's up to *me*? How refreshing. He grew nicer by the minute.

He explained why radiotherapy was the treatment of choice for me now, he told me exactly what he would do,

111

how long it would take, what sort of side-effects there might be, what would happen to my breast, what would happen to the rest of me, what to expect in the short term, what to hope for in the long term. When he'd done all that he threw in a little homily about the broader uses for radiotherapy in the therapeutic community. By the time he had finished you couldn't help wondering why everyone didn't get a dose, in the same way that school-children used to get free milk. I've always had a weakness for enthusiasts. I fell in love with him on the spot.

I could have listened to him all day, he was so keen and vigorous. Unfortunately he had to come to an end sometime, and as he did I murmured admiringly, 'That was terrific, you should have been a second-hand car salesman.'

I realize, on reflection, that might not have sounded like the compliment it was meant to be, but Howard knew exactly what I meant. He roared with laughter, causing some interest around the ward.

'Maybe so, but if I was selling second-hand cars you wouldn't be buying, would you?'

Relief. This man was on to me straight away.

Suddenly it was easy to talk and I poured out a stream of feelings and attitudes that he did his best to understand. At one point I said, 'You see, the trouble is, the way I feel about it now, I couldn't have radiotherapy whole-heartedly.'

'Well we certainly agree about that: I wouldn't want to treat you unless you did feel wholehearted about it.'

I could have kissed him.

I felt vastly better for talking to him. He has an uplifting, invigorating, healing presence; he makes you feel good just by being there. He would probably get the same results without a machine as he does with one, although being what is sometimes referred to as 'a true scientist' he wouldn't believe that for one minute. He was very worried about my decision not to have treatment, and not much mollified by my reassurance that I would go away and think about it and let him know.

'I know what you do when you "go away and think about it". You disappear without a trace for years on end.'

He had obviously read my notes pretty carefully.

112

I agreed to make an appointment to see him again after I was out of hospital. I didn't take much persuading, he was quite the most powerful and appealing person I had ever met within hospital walls. He was tough enough to withstand all the so-called pressure I was supposed to be putting on doctors by just being the sort of person I am, and kind enough to come back for more. The truth was, I couldn't bear not to see him again.

It was entirely my fault that I felt isolated and lonely in hospital. To a certain extent I had felt obliged not to see a local oncologist, but none the less it was my choice that had brought me so far from home. I watched enviously while other people in the ward enjoyed casual, pop-in visits from family and friends who were playing a part in the recovery process, making it a family affair. I hadn't dared tell half my family what was happening to me for fear they would come rushing in with recriminations and insistence that I should see reason and do as I was told. But it must be said, few as they were, my visitors were good value for money.

One of my dearest friends is married to a vet, and between the two of them they hold more esoteric and amazing views of the universe than I have ever dreamed of. In between campaigning for animal rights and lecturing to students and milking the goats, Alastair did a fifty-mile detour to visit me. He roared into the ward and took the place over. Goodness knows what he found to laugh about, but he soon had us all joining in. He wandered around, introducing himself, bringing a flush of pleasure to at least one lonely, spinster cheek. He was hugely amused by the panoramic view of the graveyard that faced us from the ward. I had wondered myself, in my more miserable moments, whether to hurl myself from the window and cut out the middle man.

'This should never have happened, I don't know what they're thinking about Up There. What a mess we must be making of everything. Never mind, all will be well. Bodies are only on loan you know.'

He said this several times and I was never quite sure what he meant by it, but it didn't matter. Every word he uttered was so remote from the language of the hospital world it was automatically inspiring, irrespective of meaning. He was not the least bit in awe of the hospital and had poked around downstairs on arrival and unearthed the chapel. Not only that, he had managed to time his visit to coincide with a service. He shepherded me out of bed and into the lift before I had time to say I was too tired.

David, Alastair and myself were the only ones taking communion. The chapel was so deeply buried in a catacomb of corridors it felt as though we were worshipping some outlawed diety in secret. It wasn't exactly the heart-beat of the hospital.

Unable to hide in the non-existent crowds, I was forced to talk to the curate who cornered me into accepting a visit from his assistant. I changed my mind about this immediately and asked sister to tell him not to come.

I automatically assumed it would be a 'him' but it was a 'her', and of course she got to me before I could stop her. Thank God. She was a great help to me. I struggled through all my feelings of failure, of having let people down, and listened to her saying firmly:

'If people choose to idolize you, that's their problem. You're punishingly hard on yourself about *your* tendency to slide into playing a role, remember that everyone else is playing that game too. You aren't responsible for what they get up to.'

It was nice to feel I wasn't responsible for everything: it was all I could do to cope with being in charge of my health.

David came to drive me home. As I eased my way tenderly into the car and protected my sore breast against the seat-belt I felt like a re-run of an old movie. How many more times was I going to do this?

There followed a few weeks of unprecedented gloom for me. I took a long time to get over the anaesthetic and my breast was pretty painful and kept me awake at night, but what haunted me most was why this had happened to me again. I always knew why I had been ill in the first place, but since then I had made a genuine attempt to face up to and work on these problems and conflicts. So why had I got it again? What was this tumour trying to tell me that the other one hadn't?

I cancelled all my patients, withdrew from the Centre,

114

thereby doubling Pat's workload, and retreated into my think tank. By which I mean I lay around all day and thought about things. It didn't take long before some painful insights started to emerge.

For one thing I had stopped looking after myself. I now had to admit that I had allowed myself to become a crazy workaholic, that all my friends who had said I was doing too much were right. I had already justified this with a set of explanations that were plausible and acceptable to me, so it was hard to see that I was making the same old mistakes again – but for different reasons. I wasn't working every hour God sent because I didn't think anyone would love me unless I did, this time I was doing it because people needed me. The effect was just the same: I lived a life that was projected entirely outwards towards others. There was hardly a moment of my time used to replenish myself.

The second thing I was beginning to understand was that, although I had learned to say 'no' a bit more often, I was still an amateur at this kind of self-defence. Perhaps there were other areas where I thought I had the problem licked, but hadn't done quite such a wonderful job as I had imagined.

So, I'd made some progress, but not enough. Was that it?

Slowly it started to dawn on me that the kind of self-knowledge and healing that I had been seeking was a process and not an event.

This was a most important revelation. I had secretly been clinging to the security of seeing all achievements as identifiable events, like riding a bike – once learned never forgotten. I certainly wanted to see my cancer as an event, because then it would be something I could put behind me, not drag around with me painfully from day to day. But perhaps recovering from cancer involved a process that went on and on, involving a whole series of healings, lots of events all strung together, blurred into each other, forming a fuzzy whole with no identifiable beginning or end. Since that was so much harder to accept it was more than likely to be right.

I went back to London to have my stitches removed. A minor surgical event that gains all its power to terrify solely because one is so helplessly dependent on the mood and performance of somebody else. It's something that can go either way. Happily I was treated gently – consistent with the way I was handled from the beginning. On my way out I was met by the young doctor who had been interested in my 'models of disease' number. We exchanged the usual pleasantries while waiting for the lift. He was having a frightfully hard time of it.

'I'm rushed off my feet actually. There's this woman on ward 5 who has to have chemotherapy, and all the chemotherapy is done on ward 7, but she's insisting on having it done on ward 5. Damned inconvenient.'

I warmed to the woman on ward 5. Fancy being tough enough to *insist* on anything where chemotherapy was concerned. Obviously she reckoned it would be easier for her to cope with it on her own ward where she knew the staff and felt secure. Easier for her, maybe, but not for my informant.

'It means I've got to go all the way up there and sort the stuff out and get the right equipment and take it all down to ward 5.'

I commiserated. 'The way some people carry on you'd think this whole building had been built especially for them, and that everyone who worked here was paid just to look after them.'

I admit this was mean of me. Really mean. But I was so thrilled at having thought of it at the time and not half way home on the train that I was unrepentant. Anyway, there may have been no need for repentance. I said it with such a sympathetic smile I'm far from certain the penny dropped, and he twittered on in the lift about all the time this was going to take and what a nuisance it was. But he did give me a funny look as I waved him goodbye.

I had learnt from the hospital that there had been some hormone dependence in the tumour as Ernesto had suspected. In view of this they had proposed that I should have my ovaries removed, either surgically or with radiotherapy treatment. I didn't fancy either course of action overmuch and decided to telephone Ernesto and see what he thought I should do.

That was definitely easier said than done. Anyone who has tried to make a quick call to Mexico will know that not only do you need shares in British Telecom to pay for it, you need

116

the undivided attention of at least one telephone operator who happens to be bilingual and is owed lots of favours by his Mexican counterpart. You also need about two days. That's how long it took us before I heard his muffled voice, hissing down the wires sounding as if he was trapped underwater in a wardrobe.

He had a great idea.

'Come and see me. I can help you, you must come and see me. This is the best thing.'

And so it might have been, but it was also out of the question. We simply didn't have the money. Or so we thought.

Somebody bought us the tickets. Two tickets to Mexico and back, so David could come with me.

I had a telephone call from an acupuncture patient. He said he had written to me and he knew some people were funny about these things and he didn't want me to take it the wrong way, so please would I understand it was what he wanted to do.

What was, for goodness' sake? Perhaps he was so fed up with me cancelling his appointments he wanted to start going to somebody else? Would that warrant such a long recital?

The letter came with a cheque for hundreds of pounds. Hundreds.

The dear gourmet friend, purveyor of delectable vegetarian-wholefood banquets arrived with casseroles of delicious comfort and a great bundle of travellers' cheques.

Anna – Alastair's wife and our dear friend – came rushing over to see me bearing her usual catholic collection of treats: home-made goat's cheese, herbal remedies, her skills as a healer and yet another cheque.

Chapter 8

To administer medicine to diseases which have already developed and to suppress revolts which have already developed is comparable to the behaviour of those persons who begin to dig a well after they have become thirsty ... would these actions not be too late?

The Yellow Emperor's Classic of Internal Medicine

It was impossible not to compare this time with the period that had preceded my departure to Germany four years before. We had been so lonely and isolated then, whereas now we were swept up in a whirlwind of concerned involvement from nearly everyone we knew. It was just as well we were, since my personal shock and confusion had left me feeling slow and lethargic. I don't think I could have organized myself to the end of the road, never mind into Mexico via America.

I had some doubts about whether I ought to go. People were coming half way across the world to see *me* at the Cancer Help Centre, what could I learn in Mexico that I didn't know already? It seemed a wild, extravagant indulgence. Maybe I was simply refusing to accept that my way of doing things just didn't work. To my surprise and annoyance someone actually telephoned me to express precisely these thoughts.

'I don't think you should go. It's a waste of time. After all, it isn't as if you haven't tried these things before. The truth of the matter is that they just don't work.'

That did it. I was going.

In a most reassuring and comforting way all my

118

uncertainty was stripped away by events. We couldn't afford to go, but people gave us money, so that ceased to be a significant factor. We had doubts but, with the exception of that one telephone call, everyone else we spoke to swept all objections aside.

'Of course you must go. You can't expect to have the whole cancer problem sewn up completely in the space of a few years. Dr Contreras is bound to be able to tell you something new.'

'We need you to go. Look at all the good that came from your going to Germany.' That was Pat of course. She always managed to turn my disasters into something important and positive.

We needed visas, and immediately Pat's daughter, Felicity, set out on our behalf to the American embassy. She returned with the rather embarrassing news that America was far from thrilled to issue a visa to one who had apparently violated UK passport regulations. It appears that it is an offence to have two valid British passports, and people who do are viewed with deep suspicion. How I had managed to obtain two passports was a mystery to me, but indeed I had. It took hours of persuasion to convince the Americans that I wasn't hell bent on a criminal career, that it was safe to let me into the Land of the Brave.

The children found it all very hard to cope with, but they were older and more experienced this time. Despite the fear and the anger that exploded on the surface, what lay unexpressed at a deeper level was the knowledge that we had survived all this before and therefore would probably survive it again. They departed to the friends who had looked after them before with the same weary anxiety that must have accompanied many a citizen into the air-raid shelters, hoping, as they had, that the flak would pass harmlessly over their heads and all would live to reminisce in years to come about the whole horrid experience.

I couldn't help feeling I had let them down.

Almost exactly four years after flying to Germany I was winging my way to Baltimore. What a way to see the world.

True to form David was having a great time. 'Darling, we're going to see southern California, it'll be lovely.

119

Everyone says it's a wonderful part of the world. Thank goodness we don't have to go to some dump in the hinterland, that would be worse.'

Quite. I made a mental note to make sure all my medical missions should be conducted in and around well-known tourist spots.

'We won't have to spend all day at the clinic, after all. It shouldn't be too difficult to cross the border back into America. We can have a good look round San Diego.'

'Do you think we could get there first before you start dragging me off to fulfil your fantasies?'

'Look Pen, I'm sorry, but how do you want me to behave? Sometimes I think you don't want to take it all too seriously.'

'Sometimes I don't.'

'But this isn't one of those times?'

'I don't know what it is.'

I wasn't very good company. Apart from anything else I also had a roaring toothache. The pressure in the plane exploding in a weak filling was a powerful, if unwelcome, distraction from my other problems.

We were on a night flight and experienced for the first time the extraordinary wonder of following the sun. Having left England in broad daylight we continued to be dazzled by brilliant sunshine for hour after hour. It was very strange, and although it was exciting, it was also rather tiring. I saw a similarity here with my own situation. I suspected that I was ahead of my time in my beliefs about the nature of illness. Although, like the perpetual sunlight, this was sometimes thrilling, it was also exhausting. I was tired of waiting for the universe to synchronize with my personal timing.

The only one in step you understand.

Flying high above the earth is a wonderful time for such metaphysical reflections. I had not the slightest doubt that one day – probably quite soon – my cranky and peculiar views would become a shared part of a common belief system. Come that day it wouldn't be necessary to search so hard and so far for understanding and guidance. Things were already better than they had been. We had lit a candle in Bristol and people were moving towards that little pinprick of light, but I still had an inoperable lump in my breast that I didn't know how to overcome. Would my problem always slightly outweigh the healing available? It was a depressing thought. What I felt I needed would come, but would it come in time for me? Remember Larkin's disappointed cry?

Sexual intercourse began
In nineteen sixty-three
(Which was rather late for me) –
Between the end of the Chatterly ban
And the Beatles' first LP.

I gazed out at the clouds and sank back with relief into a timeless feeling of detachment from the world. Maybe it would all come too late for me but there were dimensions other than this one where I belonged and would be looked after. There must be, otherwise where had all my beliefs come from? They existed somewhere, even if everyone else hadn't cottoned on to them yet. I felt like a visitor from another planet and cheered up immediately. I reached out my hand to touch David, 'I'm sorry I snapped at you. You're right, we'll probably have a lovely time.'

'Of course we will. We might even get up to Los Angeles – now that *would* be something ...'

Typical. Given half a chance he always pushes his luck. But how could I dare to criticize him? Without him my bleached bones would have been swept up years later from the floor of Baltimore airport, where I lay exhausted in the transit lounge. He had slotted into his role of confident explorer as if he had spent half his life jet-setting around the world. He has the knack of travelling. He always has small coins in foreign currency for slot machines, and is the envy of all the other exhausted travellers who stand around gazing wistfully at pictures of steaming cups of coffee, clutching useless $100 bills. He de-bugs the unfamiliar intricacies of different telephone systems in seconds, and within hours is explaining the bus timetable to people who have lived on the route all their lives.

The second leg of the journey took us across America to San Diego. We were treated to our first experience of the chummy, casual Californian style by our pilot who chattered over the tannoy.

'Hello folks, this is Captain Warbangerwatsit.' (They all seemed to have very funny names.) 'As soon as my co-pilot has finished winding up the rubber bands we shall be flying terribly high up in the air, lots of thousands of feet up, no doubt about it. And while you're all having a great time watching the in-flight movie we'll be trying to dodge the worst of the bumpy bits. Rumour has it there's a bit of turbulance out there, but don't worry about a thing, we've both had hours of practice on the simulator.'

This was all very entertaining, but was it quite what I wanted from an airline pilot? I comforted myself with the thought that you'd have to be very confident and sure of yourself to clown around in this way.

'Me again folks. Just to add a little interest to your flight we are offering a prize of two bottles of best California wine to the person who can guess how many gallons of fuel we shall use to fly from here to our halfway point.'

For one heart-stopping moment I waited for him to add that he'd like to have our answers as soon as possible in order to make sure he'd put enough petrol in the tanks. He didn't.

Before the stewards even came around with the competition forms David was scribbling calculations on the back of an envelope and muttering about prevailing winds.

Of course he won. Not only that, his figure was short by a mere four gallons. The steward was visibly impressed, said nobody had ever been so close before, except a small boy who had made a wild guess, but that didn't cut any icy with the professionals. Obviously David knew what he was about. Had he done any flying before? I wondered whether Warbangerwatsit-Biggles up at the sharp end might be sounding him out to lend a hand if the going got rough in the bumpy bits. Mercifully it was a smooth and uneventful flight.

When we finally landed at San Diego David had a great time playing around with a glittering, colourful display of advertisements for hotels that was attached to a free 'phone-in-for-further-details' scheme.

There was no point in trying to get to Mexico that night since it was already ten o'clock local time, so we made our weary way to the nearest cheap hotel. I was wide awake at four in the morning. Exhausted, but not sleepy, my mind was buzzing with questions about why I had come, what I thought I would gain from it, what were the children doing now, would we be able to contact Ernesto in the morning. He knew we were coming, but he didn't know when. Obviously there is a fixed quota on successful telephone calls from the UK to Mexico, and we had used ours up. Despite hours of trying we had failed to make contact about specific times and dates. Supposing he wasn't there? What if he had gone on holiday?

To my horror that was exactly what he had done. The following day was Sunday, and the woman we spoke to at the Clínico del Mar said Dr Contreras was away for a few days, but would be back on Monday. We decided to wait and go down to Tijuana the following day. This left us free to wander around San Diego for the day. David was off in a flash. He borrowed a map from the receptionist and worked out an itinerary before we had finished breakfast.

By midday we had walked what felt like the entire length of the waterside.

'We're very lucky to have the chance to do this,' he insisted. 'It's just the thing to get our blood circulating after sitting down in that plane for so long.' It's so annoying being married to someone who's always right. No doubt he feels the same.

But it was a lovely day. A warm, sunny, friendly day. Everyone seemed keen for us to enjoy ourselves.

'Have a nice day,' smiled the passing promenaders. 'Have a nice day,' gasped the overtaking joggers. 'Have a nice day,' puffed the swerving cyclists. How could we do anything but.

Another restless night in the hotel and then off to Mexico. No need for me to explain that most people hired cars. Air-conditioned cars driven by people who knew the ropes, who crossed forth and back across the border all the time, offering door to door service. No need for me to explain that we didn't do this. We had all the fun of humping our luggage to the bus stop and taking up twice the number of seats we had paid for. Then the thrill of the Santa Fe railway and its bone-shaking seats, to be followed by a long, hot and uncomfortable wait at the border for a car to take us where we wanted to go. David should have done his travelling with Livingstone or E M Forster at the very least. I fear I rather cramped his style, but I need not have worried. Anyone who is thrilled with himself for knowing to the nearest minute what time the bus will come, and who gets a buzz from working out the vagaries of the ticket machine is having an impenetrably happy time. He was a pleasure to be with. If I occasionally felt like a native bearer shuffling along behind, well, that was my problem.

Nobody at the clinic seemed to have any idea who we were, and there was no sign of Ernesto. We lay on the bed in our room and tried to sort out our impressions.

Nothing was as I had expected it to be. For a start, I was really shocked at the poverty and squalor in Mexico. This was highlighted, of course, by the stunning contrast with America. San Diego is a pretty, clean and affluent town, with many attractive parks and architectural features. It was a shock to travel only a few miles from there and find oneself in a place full of makeshift shacks and pot-holed roads, with overspilt rubbish blowing around in the dust. What made it even more shocking was the fact that this was likely to be one of the better parts of the country. I had to admit to myself that I had always had a romantic and sentimental vision of Mexico that had something to do with beautiful people who were carefree and sang a lot. Obviously I'd been watching too many Westerns. These people were beautiful all right, but they were poor. Grindingly poor. I couldn't imagine them feeling carefree or having much to sing about. The Clínico del Mar was the most prosperous looking place for miles around.

In Ernesto's absence I was examined by another young Mexican doctor who made copious notes. He was accompanied by an American girl, also a doctor, and interested in the work of the clinic. She was very small and slight and, I learned later, rather shy. Whenever she caught my eye she smiled at me. I wondered what she was making of my case history. She probably thought I was tough enough to cope with all this by now, but I was feeling thoroughly miserable and hating every minute of it. Why did I subject myself to these things – unfamiliar places, foreign voices and faces? To make matters worse I had to have an internal examination. I was wondering if I could bear this when she slipped her warm hand under the blanket and squeezed mine. Such a sweet, small gesture. It was enough. Knowing that she empathized, that she cared enough to show me that she too would feel rotten and miserable in such a circumstance, knowing that strengthened me. Returning the pressure of her hand I felt the comfort of feeling I was not alone.

We wandered around the clinic picking up leaflets, talking to other patients, trying to find out what it was all about. This was a lot easier than the same effort in Germany. For a start we were talking the same language, and for another thing Ernesto was using many techniques that were familiar. Dr Contreras is the ultimate holistic practitioner. He has built a hospital a few miles away from the clinic where patients who need to, undergo surgery and have radiotherapy or chemotherapy. Obviously this aspect of his work was easy to understand and he was justifiably proud of his hospital. But his long experience with cancer had shown him that this was not enough. Patients needed more than this. So, in addition to his medical and surgical facilities he has nutritionists who talk about food, psychologists who unravel your emotional knots, enthusiasts who explain coffee enemas, and a constant supply of amygdalin.

This is the most controversial aspect of his therapy. Amygdalin is extracted from apricot kernels and is a substance absolutely guaranteed to infuriate most conservative medics the world over. Ernesto is a great believer in its use as part of a cancer control regime, and nearly everyone who visits his clinic will receive high doses of this substance, intravenously, every day. They will also have Bible study groups and sessions of chorus singing and services in the beautiful pink church he has built just around the corner. Like I said, the ultimate holistic practitioner.

He returned from his holiday bubbling with delight at seeing us again. He read carefully through my notes and examined me again.

'This is very strange that this area is proved to be malignant. It does not feel like a typical malignancy, but we must believe now that it is and act accordingly. Tell me what they say in England that you should do?'

I told him. And not just the broad outline either, not just scrappy little bits of information wrestled from the reluctant lips of consultants free with remarks like, 'If I told you, you wouldn't understand.' No, I was now in the hands of the inimitable Dr Howard who had come up trumps again. In between leaving the hospital and flying out to Mexico I had been back to see him. He asked me if I had decided what to do about the radiotheraphy treatment and listened patiently as I explained about the possibility of going to see Dr Contreras.

'I think that's probably a good idea. It obviously means a lot to you and that's important. Just promise you'll come and see me as soon as you get back.'

I could hardly believe my ears. Emboldened, I asked if he would explain again just what he had in mind for radiotherapy treatment so I could tell Dr Contreras.

'Once a day, five days a week for six weeks.'

'Yes, I see, thank you. But what does that actually mean? Are there different doses? How do you measure radio-therapy – is it in rads? Could you tell me how many rads I'll have to have?'

He did look a bit taken aback by that but, would you believe it, he told me. Not only that, he wrote it all down on a piece of paper. It was this script that I slid across the desk to Ernesto. He read it slowly and then said,

'This is very sensitive treatment. If ever you must have radiotherapy, you should have it from this man.'

It was worth flying half way round the world just to hear that.

'They want to radiate my ovaries too because of the oestrogen receptors in the tumour – but I really don't want that, it seems so crude and violent. It just doesn't seem right to me.'

Ernesto heard me out.

'Well this is one way, and of course surgery is another, but there is always tamoxifen. This is a drug that acts on oestrogens. It is widely used in these circumstances.'

'Dr Howard says that's not as good.'

'He may be right. This is a complex area. Nobody knows for certain what is best, but if you are wishing to avoid extreme measures, it may be good for you. Think about it. In the meantime I shall discuss your case with my colleagues here. I have certain opinions, but I must see also what they think. You must have the benefit of all our knowledge. In a few days I will tell you what our conference concludes.'

He closed my file and dropped it on the desk. Standing up with a beaming smile he held his arms out to us both. 'We must pray that God will help us find His way for you. And now I shall take you to eat, Rita is waiting for us.' With that he hung up his white coat and swept us off to Tijuana for lunch.

The few days that we had spent wandering around the clinic had revealed to me that Ernesto's ideas about diets for cancer patients were a lot more relaxed and liberal than my own. It is true that he issued everyone with a diet sheet and that the principles were the same in broad outline as Issels' and others – no animal protein, no salt, sugar, preservatives, low fat. But the kitchen in the clinic cafeteria served the most delicious wholewheat brownies and other tempting eggy/cheesy things that would have raised a fussier eyebrow. When we talked about this later he explained.

'People can only cope with just so much. They will do their best, but if we make it too hard for them they will give up altogether.'

Nevertheless I was just a little startled when he ushered us into an enormous Chinese restaurant. A vast, glittering emporium that served a memorable meal well lashed with monosodium glutamate.

For the next couple of days I tottered around having blood tests and keeping appointments while my body clock slowly recovered from the insult of the jet-lag. David and I both faithfully attended all the talks and classes – biblical and biological – but there was little here that was new to us. We were guarded in what we said to each other, neither wanting to admit to being disappointed, but feelings of uncertainty about having come hovered around us, and we gave in to a sorry combination of depression and tiredness. I was delighted to have had Ernesto's confirmation of my faith in

Dr Howard's skill and sensitivity, but I was not blind to the fact that I could have established this by letter. This, and the fact that other patients at the clinic were using me as a useful fount of knowledge and experience, made the whole extravagance of flying half way around the world a bit *de trop*. I recognized in this journey some of the 'silver bullet' syndrome: a frantic attempt to find an answer to the problem that lay 'out there' rather than 'in here'. How strange that I could realize the foolishness of this way of dealing with the problem and yet still be vulnerable to it lure.

From time to time I eyed with longing David's prize bottles of California wine. These had been humped from planes to buses to trams to taxis, and were now coming nicely to the boil in the corner of our hot little room. But, unlike Issels, wine was no part of Ernesto's plan. He and his family were strictly teetotal. Not surprising in view of the dreadful influence of alcohol in the poorer parts of Mexican society. This made our bottles in the wardrobe look decidedly seedy. Even so, there were times when I thought a few hours of woozy oblivion would have been very welcome, and I resisted only because I knew that once I started on that particular temptation I should be in real trouble.

By the middle of our first week there we were both feeling a bit weary and jaded with the whole cancer business, and in this frame of mind we wandered along to Ernesto's startling, sugar-pink church for an evening bible class. A dozen or so patients sat awkwardly in the front pews waiting for their healer-priest. Ernesto arrived and instructed us all to read a verse of his chosen passage. I watched and listened while people who had never held a sacred text of any sort in their hands, never mind read aloud from one, found their places and read out their verses. Admittedly there was a young Methodist minister there and a few others who knew the ropes, but the atheists, the agnostics, the 'don't knows', all seemed quite happy about it as well.

Ernesto drew all the meaning and comfort he could from the scriptures so precious to him and offered this to his little band of suffering souls, just as he had earlier that day given to their bodies his best interpretation and application of his medical skills. When he had finished he invited us to stay for the mid-week service of praise that was about to start in the church.

A few of us decided to do this and watched curiously as the benches filled up with the participants of all the other bible classes that had been taking place in various rooms around the building. Every generation was represented: youngsters dashed about knocking things over and slamming doors, teenagers solemnly tuned their guitars, old people sat down softly with a sigh. Within minutes the place was packed. Someone elected to take the microphone and welcome us all – in Spanish of course – and the service was under way.

How can I describe it? My Spanish is about as good as my German – which means I didn't understand a word that was being said or sung, but this really didn't matter at all. Ernesto played the organ, the children crouched with lip-moving intensity over their instruments, the great Latin temperament of the congregation raised its arms in adoration of its Lord, and the Holy Spirit whistled like a wind around the church. It was the most wonderful experience of God that I had ever known.

I wondered briefly how David was responding to this. After all, the inhibitions of my religious background – Cornish Methodists and Welsh Baptists don't go in for this swaying about, arm waving and getting carried away – were as nothing to those of a nice Jewish boy from West Hampstead. I didn't wonder for long of course, because this kind of experience transcends all such trivia; he was swept up as I was, as we all were, in the wonder of the presence of God.

Such experiences are timeless and I have no idea for how long we were part of that oneness. Reason suggests that the service must have lasted about an hour, but its influence will last for ever.

The difficulty with all belief systems, and Christianity is no exception to this, is to get them out of your head and into action. From the intellectual to the actual. Why we should find this almost universally hard to do I do not fully understand, but I know it is a stumbling block for many people. Perhaps it's all wrapped up with the stiff-upper-lip department of the great British public school tradition. For years we have been taught specifically not to show our feelings, even to go so far as to suppress them if necessary. The justification for all this was that the expression of emotions and feelings would automatically lead to loss of control. I am increasingly of the view that the reverse is true: I think the more we are in touch with our emotions the more we understand them and know what they feel like. Only then can we hope to exercise any control over them. But of course, in order to achieve this, we have to let go occasionally. For me, this was just such an occasion. That service of prayer and praise didn't belong in the world of the intellect, it belonged in the world of responsiveness. For that reason it is bound to defy my efforts to describe it. For a brief time my normal boundaries were swept away and I could know God without the restrictions that my culture, religion, nature and style would usually impose. This allowed me to perceive Him in a great, sweeping wave of Kundalini, to know that this God was within me, part of me, part of the people I was with, the living spirit of the whole created universe, unaffected by our limited realities, always there, not bargaining with us, just waiting for us to wake up to Him.

Not surprisingly, I felt a lot better for this.

We spent the rest of the evening eating cakes and drinking tea with Ernesto and Rita, meeting other members of their family. One of Ernesto's sons, Paco, is also a doctor. A highly qualified surgeon, he trained in Vienna and chose to come back and support his father's work in Tijuana. He is married to a beautiful girl, has an exquisite little daughter, a magnificent new Porsche, and the best looks I've ever encountered outside the cinema. I watched while he took a late phone call from the hospital. Bouncing his baby on his hip he frowned in concentration. While she tugged at his hair and pulled at the telephone he agreed the situation was not serious, but the patient was in distress, he would come. He explained this to us with a shrug and a smile and was gone; well on the way to being a Gentle Giant in his own right. So far Ernesto qualifies as the gentlest giant of them all, but Paco will have to be the best looking.

Conversation was about Ernesto's brother, whose ruby wedding celebrations were scheduled to take place that weekend. It was generally agreed that Ernesto and Rita should attend, a decision that left me feeling very miserable. The party was to be in Mexico City and required that they should both be away for several days. The very days during which I was meant to have started my tamoxifen treatment, a time when I was keen to have Ernesto on hand.

You may wonder why the initiation of a simple oestrogen-control therapy should have been such a big deal for me. Women in their millions are taking it all the time, but as usual I had managed to turn the whole thing into a drama. For one thing, I was acknowledging that there was a place for a bit of interventionist therapy in my programme, which until that time was heavily biased towards internal transformation without external pressure. So taking these tablets was quite a big psychological step. In addition to this I had, of course, read up all I could about the possible side effects and had formed a frightening picture of myself, bent double with stomach cramps and well into the menopause, all within the space of a few days. The very days during which Ernesto was threatening to disport himself in Mexico. Imagine my delight when he suggested we should come too.

'We would love you to come. You can see so much in Mexico City. My sister will be pleased for you to stay in her house. You will not need money – just for the plane ticket. Please come.'

Anna and Alastair had given us almost the exact fare. Certain that they would have considered a climb up the Great Pyramid of the Sun a vastly more healing experience than kicking around Tijuana, we agreed to go.

We didn't need much persuading because David in particular had been stir crazy almost from the moment of arrival. The Centro Clínico del Mar is situated on the outskirts of Tijuana and the immediate surroundings had little to offer. In Germany, the RingbergKlinik was within a few minutes of beautiful walking country, whereas it didn't look to me as though anybody did much walking in our Mexican environment. Everyone seemed to scream around the place in the shattered wrecks of old Fords or Buicks, bumpers crashing along the ground, leaving a fine trail of sparks and rust in their wake. The roads around the clinic

131

looked and sounded like a scrap heap that had magically come to life. Even if you weren't flattened by one of these hooting, squealing resurrected wonders, or stunned by a high-flying hub-cap, there wasn't really anywhere to go in the immediate vicinity. This didn't suit David at all.

'I don't think I can stand this much longer. I've got to get some exercise. There must be a way down to the beach somewhere – I'm going for a run.'

He dodged off across the main road in his Adidas shorts to a cacophony of encouraging hoots and toots, making his own personal contribution to the 'mad dogs and Englishmen' syndrome.

He returned triumphant.

Yes, he had found a way down to the beach. No, it wasn't really very nice, it looked as though the promenade had collapsed at some time and there was rather a lot of broken concrete lying around. Well, yes, rather a lot of rubbish too, but if you went further down the coast there was a beautiful place, a kind of park. Most attractive and clean, very tidy and well-cared for. It was odd though, because there didn't seem to be an obvious way in, but it didn't matter because someone had broken down the fence in a most convenient place and he had run through there. So, it was all a big success if you didn't mind the tacky start, and was I coming next time? No thanks. Only because I hadn't packed my shorts, of course.

Lies all lies. I hate jogging, and when you've got cancer you don't worry overmuch about heart disease. The early morning runs were a little treat he could have all to himself. In any event they were not destined to last very long. His enthusiastic description of his sporting achievements were greeted with a grasp of horror by Rita.

'You mustn't do that! You are running across the border. Every day you are running in and out of America. You could get arrested for this.'

That explained the beautiful park with the broken down fence.

Apparently some other poor innocent doing the same thing had been picked up by the border patrol. Since, quite understandably, he wasn't carrying his passport in his sweatshirt it took several days for him to prove he was who he said he was. Several days which he spent in a Mexican prison.

'You'd better come with us to Mexico City, it's safer.'

It seemed like a good idea for lots of reasons, and of course the glint was back in David's eye.

'This is fantastic. Who would have thought we'd ever get to Mexico City. I can't believe our good luck. And to be staying with a family too – it's not like having to go as a tourist – what an opportunity ...'.

I was quite well adjusted to my role of tour operator *extraordinaire* by now and actually felt very excited about the whole idea myself. David darted off to get tickets in Tijuana while I continued to apply myself, rather half-heartedly, to the schedule of appointments I had at the clinic. One of these was with the psychologist.

Ernesto's system required you to pay for everything in advance at the office and you were then given a ticket telling you where and when to present yourself. Nothing could have been a more striking contrast to the systematic, crisp structure of the RingbergKlinik in Germany where occasionally the routine could feel a bit heartless, or even rather intimidating. Here you were given an appointment time that was optimistically calculated to the nearest minute and then you settled yourself outside the appropriate room and proceeded to wait for hours on end. The first time this happened to me I ran the whole gamut of responses: from disbelief to irritation, on to rage, and finally settling with righteous indignation. By the time I was eventually ushered, hours late, into the consulting room by a smiling, totally unrepentent Mexican my blood pressure had doubled. Fortunately for me I adapted very quickly to this rather unpredictable, fluid way of doing things, and within days long years of conscientious time-keeping lay in a peaceful heap. The clinic ran on a binary time system: 'American' time for when it really mattered, 'Mexican' time for when it really didn't.

The psychologist was a gentle, mild man in his thirties. He was Mexican and, like Paco, had beautiful black eyes. He sat watching me with these for an inordinately long time, slowly sifting through my notes without looking at them. I wondered whether I was meant to kick off. If so, what in the world should I say? At last he tapped my notes and sighed, 'You work very hard. You seem a very important person, seeing many patients for acupuncture, working in your cancer clinic, and also you have three children. This is a lot for one person to do, even a strong healthy person. Tell me one thing: when do you play?'

Play! When indeed. I was by now embarrassingly aware of my tendency to turn all my pleasure and leisure activities into The Week's Good Cause, and then wonder why they weren't fun any more.

He sighed again. I couldn't tell if he was bored or broken-hearted.

'In every day there are twenty-four hours. I think it is good for you to work maybe eight of these hours, then you must sleep also, another eight. Now this is the most important thing – for the other eight hours you should play.'

He questioned me gently about the things I love to do – like playing the violin.

'How often do you play?'

I didn't like to say I'd spent more time out in the corridor waiting for him than I had managed in torturing my favourite Telemann pieces. Suddenly I wanted to cry for the loss of it all. The enthusiasm, the messing about, the not having to be purposeful or productive or important. Why couldn't I hang on to this side of myself? Why did I insist on this long, slow suicide of over-achieving?

There was no point in prolonging the interview. I agreed to come again and rose to leave.

'One more thing. Do you eat candy?'

With a rash of indignation, knowing that this at least I could get right, I retorted, 'No, of course not. I never eat things like that – I'm very careful about what I eat.'

Another sigh. 'No, I thought not. You should eat more candy. Be kind to yourself, don't be so stiff and hard. Eat more candy.'

Feeling more like Alice in Wonderland than ever I promised to think about it.

This simple encounter had a deep effect on me although I was not aware of this at the time. As soon as the door had closed behind me I was telling myself I hadn't had my money's worth and I stomped back to my room in a graceless humour. Nevertheless it was abundantly clear to me that, apart from the intravenous amygdalin, Ernesto's metabolic therapy could not offer me anything new, and it was obvious that I would do well to pursue what he had to offer in the mind and spirit departments.

I decided to avail myself of the services of another psychologist who attended the clinic for one day a week, temporarily absenting himself from some kind of holistic healing centre in San Diego. He was everything a Southern Californian psychoanalyst should be: crinkly-eyed and smily, checking your Christian name with a bone-crunching handshake, and free with phrases like 'Where you're at' ..., 'Where you're coming from' ..., 'the thrust of our relationship this afternoon' ..., and so on.

I thought I'd like to try a taste of this and booked myself in for an hour. Poor chap. He tried a mild sortie along the lines of, 'Let's see what this cancer is saying to you. What lies behind it ...' and I shot him down in flames. I'd done all that. I'd panned away at my disease in precisely this fashion for years, and admittedly there were still a few stubborn little stones left – about a tendency to resist pleasure and embrace exertion – but why wasn't I reaping the rewards of all my other, slightly more successful efforts? If my psyche was so desperate to tell me things about myself, why did it only seem to show an interest in my failures? There were things that I'd dealt with over the years that had gone really well. I was no longer a self-pitying martyr: not resentful; making much more honest and satisfying relationships; not so fearful; more aware. How about a pat on the back for being a good girl instead of a lump in the breast for not being quite good enough?

As you can see I hadn't progressed far from the days of 'rewards and fairies', but I was ready to move, and this particular man enabled me to do it. Very wisely he made a habit of taping all his interviews so I have a record of every word that passed between us. Our conversation is punctuated by a lot of squeaky noises which came from the leather chairs, and some extremely long silences which came from me being too emotional to speak. I was in the hands of an expert. Within minutes he knew enough about me to explain his approach and he led me into areas that I had only flirted with before, but never really explored. Actually it isn't fair to say he led me, he accompanied me, he allowed me and encouraged me. He knew that the answers to my dilemmas would come from me and not from him, so he actually said very little, but what he did say was interesting. When I expostulated that my first run-in with cancer as a psychosocial drama had been easy because my problems were so obvious, sticking up like icebergs, but this time it was difficult because I couldn't see clearly where the obstacles lay, he said, 'That's because you're a different person now. You've changed quite a bit, Penny, you aren't the same person now that you were then. This experience may require quite different processes from you.'

So, he wasn't suggesting that I had 'gone wrong' somewhere, but that I had moved on, and should perhaps be operating in a different area, not obsessively picking over the remains of the last one.

Of course, of course – processes, not events. I'd wondered about this in hospital, a few weeks earlier, when trying to analyse the feelings of unease I had about doing 'more of the same'. The thought that had been nibbling away at me then was the idea of recovery and personal development being a process, and therefore subject to change. Thus it was that the thought of a stricter diet, more hours spent in meditation and so on seemed a rather naïve response. Equally unproductive was the thought that I should rehash my personality in some way. I wanted to go beyond all this.

'Sure you do, and you have. You've run through quite a few therapists in your time, Penny. Josef Issels, Ainslie Meares and Contreras – these people are world-famous, household names to us, but for you they are familiar, even friends. You embrace them when you meet, they know you by name. And yet none of them has satisfied you, you break away from them, taking something of what they have to offer, but never accepting totally what they say. Every time you do this you make yourself harder to reach, but there is a sense in which this is a conscious choice on your part. I think

136

you are quite deliberately seeking a different kind of wisdom, a different kind of belonging. You are so close, maybe soon you will just be able to dip your hand into the stream of consciousness ...'

That was a thought to be reckoned with. But in the meantime should I dip my hand into the medical bag and make use of what they had to offer? We talked about my built-in antipathy to this way of resolving disease. I realized, to my surprise, that I felt more detached about that possible course of action than I ever had before. Once I had been convinced that any introduction of outside chemical or surgical agents would reduce my hold on my potential for inner change, but now I knew that nothing would deflect me from that path. I had gone too far along this particular track to lose my way on it. For the first time in years I saw that I could pick and choose across the board, using whatever aids I felt were appropriate to keeping me comfortable or alive, without feeling threatened, or some kind of failure. The inner acceptance of this possibility was a real letting go for me and I felt positively light-headed as a result.

Finally he asked me, 'What is it, Penny, that you are trying to do?'

I haven't listened to this tape very often, but whenever I do I feel very strange when I hear this part. There is a silence stretching into minutes, followed by the sound of my voice saying very slowly: 'I want to transcend ... yes ... that's what I want to do ... I want to transcend.'

Half an hour later, lying on my bed and listening to the tape, I couldn't believe my ears. What on earth was I saying? Transcend! What did I mean 'transcend'? It was like listening to the voice of my own subconscious and then trying to understand the meaning of it with my consciousness. Precisely what I had been struggling to do for a long time. All those 'altered states of consciousness' exercises with Max Cade, trying to get in touch with my intuitive self, that had been the beginning, but the translation of what is picked up in this way on to an active level of performance – that was the tricky bit. But I felt closer than I ever had before to making sense of these messages. It was rather strange I had to admit, but it was also exciting and wonderful and full of

137

interest and new potential and I was suddenly terribly glad that I had come.

More glad than ever when I found myself winging my way over vast, uninhabited tracts of Mexican desert on my way to one of the most interesting cities in the world. I was in just the right mood for another aeroplane journey.

While it had been the ineffable (and, thankfully, prolific) Anthony Powell who had seen me through my stay in Germany, it was Doris Lessing I had brought with me this time. Airborne between Tijuana and Zacatecas I read in *The Sirian Experiments*

> This deviant individual in [the] group – he or she has been unquestioningly and happily conformingly part of this group, and then new ideas creep in. Where do they come from ... Now her mind holds other ideas. Of what whole is she now a part? Of what invisible whole?

It gave me a slight frisson of excitement reading this so soon after having had such similar thoughts on the flight from England. The knowledge that someone could so succinctly, almost casually, express my feelings was pleasantly comforting, but it also had the effect of making my agonies over why I didn't seem to fit in anywhere look a bit pedantic. The fact was, I belonged somewhere. I lay back and indulged in a little speculation about who my fellow-travellers might be and how I might make contact with them.

Down to earth with a bumpy landing at Mexico City. A wet, humid evening, flashing lights, weaving cars, all esoteric speculations wiped out by much more human needs for food and rest. Both supplied with quiet generosity by Ernesto's sister who turned out to be captivatingly lovely. She had a beautiful, tranquil face that seemed to be smiling, even in repose. She lived, with her husband, in an elegant house with cool marble floors, and immediately offered to show us to our room. She preceded us up the stairs, her delicate hands fluttering sensitively around her as she checked her safe passage. She was almost totally blind. Was it two nights, or three, that we spent in her home? I know it was a short time, and shorter still was the time I actually spent in her company, but I can recall very clearly the contact that we had together.

I was shocked by her peaceful tolerance of her blindness because I feared my own response to such a challenge would fall far short of hers. She in turn felt a sympathy for me that seemed incongruous coming from her. In short, we were both well adjusted to our own portion of suffering and somewhat in awe of each other. We sat together on my bed one evening and laughed about this. It certainly gave me something to think about.

Her condition was irreversible, the slow fading of her remaining light an inexorable process. She was at peace with this because she had accepted it. Would I be more peaceful if I could accept my cancer in the same way? But if I did, then wasn't that just giving up? This was certainly the way I had always thought until now, but reflecting on her I wondered if I had not muddled together a perfectly reasonable objection to disease with a more subtle deep-seated reluctance to admit to my own mortality. I felt I saw in this lovely woman a person who had not confused suffering with mortality, and consequently was making a mighty fine job of coping with both.

I was full of these thoughts the following morning when Ernesto and Rita plunged us into a day of sightseeing. Now the roles were reversed, this time they showed us their treasures while we responded with varying degrees of awe, amazement and exhaustion. They knew we were very keen to see the pyramids and, after a tasty lunch of tacos made our way to the site.

Anywhere else and such a phenomenal monument would have been cluttered with ringroads, officious parking attendants, expensive turnstiles and fast food cafés. Instead these wonders rose up from a barren, jejune landscape, surrounded only by the scrappy little stalls of dusky sellers of glittery artefacts. The warm air carried the haunting sounds of soft notes blown through crude clay pipes which the bare-footed children were trying to sell. We brought one home, as if by such a gesture we could recapture the charm of that atmosphere, but such things do not belong in middle-class suburban homes, and, most appropriately, it fell to pieces.

Ernesto and Rita waited gratefully in the shade while we set out to climb to the top. There is more than one pyramid on this site, but we chose the Great Pyramid of the Sun and from the summit looked across at its partner, the Great Pyramid of the Moon, and, in between, the Avenue of the Dead. The puzzling inconsistencies of the guidebook suggest that knowledge of what actually went on here is pretty speculative, but who needs to know? It was enough to stand there in awe of the people who had put together such a place. The magnificent Avenue of the Dead marching off into the distance suggested that they had their views about mortality well sewn up. Standing there with the breeze on my face, gazing out across the plains, I felt the first stirrings of true acceptance in myself. This life is just a temporary gift, a concept we always find difficult to learn – a loan. Children struggle with this: 'Is this mine to keep, or do I have to give it back?'

You have to give it back sooner or later, cancer or no cancer. Better to concentrate on what you do with it than speculate on how to keep it. With this decidedly self-improving notion in my head we then embarked upon the descent, which was so precipitous and insecure I immediately abandoned such thoughts in favour of arriving at the bottom as just another tourist, and not a candidate for the burial chambers.

The fortieth wedding celebrations went off in style, with David and myself trying unsuccessfully to take a back seat and ending up as guests of honour, overwhelmed by typical Mexican hospitality.

On the flight back to Tijuana I decided to take the tamoxifen tablets.

By the middle of the following week Ernesto called us into his office to discuss the case conference he and his colleagues had completed about me. In the light of the results of a battery of tests they had discussed the various options available to me: removal or irradiation of the ovaries; radiation to the breast itself. They knew my preference was not to do any of these things and they too tended to share this view. They felt that I should continue with the amygdalin injections and various other therapies, while watching very carefully to see if changes were taking place that might indicate that things were getting out of hand and requiring more aggressive intervention. I was delighted to hear this but nervous about such crucial self-monitoring. Would Dr Howard be prepared to do this for me? I knew I lacked the detachment to do it properly for myself.

It was time to go home and ask him.

I felt a bit sheepish on my return from Mexico. It is true that I had made what was for me the monumentous decision to take tamofixen, but this was hardly something to make a song and dance about. Apart from that and the amygdalin injections I had made very few changes to the programme I had been following before. In contrast, I had staggered back from Germany weighted down with whole cases full of pills and potions and drenches and rubs, and full of defiant talk about 'whole body therapy' which had the appeal of novelty then, but was looking decidedly old hat by now. In short, there was very little to show for my visit, although, inwardly I felt I had gained a lot.

Dr Howard greeted me enthusiastically and launched into a discussion about Mexico, a country he seemed to know very well. He was interested in what Ernesto had said, pleased at the evaluation of his proposed radiotherapy treatment, disappointed that I was still of a mind not to have it.

'You're taking such a risk, I really do wish I could persuade you.'

'Well, if anyone could, you could, but please don't try. Could you just measure the lump and examine me and then keep a record of how things are going? I know I'll reconsider quickly enough if it gets bigger, or starts to spread.'

Crunch time for Dr Howard. Exactly what I had asked my GP to do when the first lump appeared and he had flatly refused.

'All right, if that's what you want I'll do my best. But you must understand something. I'm not in the habit of doing this, in fact I've never done anything quite like it before. I'll do the best I can, but I can't guarantee that the first sign of trouble will be local to the breast or the axilla. By leaving an active cancer untreated we run the risk of it metastasizing immediately to the lungs or the ribs, or anywhere. If that happens we'll have lost the advantage we have now.'

He said something, rather gruffly, to the effect that if I was brave enough to cope with the situation, he ought to have the courage to do his bit.

Thus we began a ritual that continues to this day.

Despite my jaundiced views about many medical matters, I still retained at this time a touching faith in the wonders of high technology. I had a mental picture of measurements being taken with sensitive callipers capable of making microscopic readings which could be expressed as a sixteen figure decimal number. I was a bit surprised when Dr Howard whipped a plastic, six-inch ruler from his top pocket and proceeded to juggle this around my lumps and bumps.

'I'm glad to see you're taking this seriously,' I murmured.

'Oh, it's very important to be accurate. I insist on all my students using rulers.'

I was most relieved. It must be one up from the naked eye.

We finally agreed on the shape and dimensions of my hilly terrain. Little drawings and numbers were duly noted in my file and I started to feel confident.

'Come and see me soon. Two weeks if possible, three at the most.'

Dr Howard obviously wasn't very confident. Clearly he expected the situation to deteriorate, and to do so quickly. I went home pretending to be a lot more sure of myself than I really was, and feeling thoroughly fed up that nobody else ever thought to look on the bright side, if only for therapeutic reasons.

The next few months were unmitigatingly awful. I wasn't working so I had nothing to distract me from obsessional introspection. My doctor refused to give me the amygdalin injections, as I had known he would, and I had to enlist as a 'temporary resident' with someone more sympathetic. This was a doctor a few miles from my home who felt that to refuse treatment of any sort, however cranky, for a disease which no right-minded person could claim as curable was not in the true Hippocratic spirit. He was lovely, but his partners would make no exceptions to their rules about only taking local patients, so my contact with him was brief. Briefer than

I had intended because I started to have a few funny reactions to the injections. I discovered that other people had also experienced this and decided to stop at once. Ernesto prepares all his own amygdalin, but import regulations made it impossible for me to get supplies from him, and I felt I would be mad to take risks.

The therapy I had brought back from Mexico was now pared down even thinner. Uneasily I leaned into the fact that recovery was more and more up to me and, finally, more than five years after my original diagnosis, I sank into depression.

I became seriously and profoundly and pathetically depressed.

This had not happened to me before. I had been frightened, angry, confused and miserable before, but had never known this unremitting paleness that drifted round me like an undefinable cloud. I lay around the house all day eating and sleeping and trying not to be too awful to live with. I put on weight, which made me feel even worse, and was unfairly annoyed when Dr Howard exclaimed that this was a good sign. Ironically enough, he was cautiously pleased. I went back as promised within a few weeks, and then again a short time after that. He did his trick with the six-inch ruler, chewed his cheeks a bit and pronounced that nothing seemed to be happening.

'Of course, we must see this as a positive sign. After all, one would expect it to be getting worse, so the fact that it doesn't appear to be changing means you are effecting some degree of control. Of course I still wish you'd have the radio-therapy ...'

Now that he had become so encouraging I no longer had ears to hear it.

I trailed off miserably to visit Ludi Howe. A counsellor at the Centre, she had been helpful to me on occasions.

'Don't give me all this para-psychology, Ludi, I need something tougher than that.'

'Do you, do you ... Yes, well perhaps you should consider taking a look at the more directly spiritual path. I have a contact that might be helpful to you.'

That night I found myself telephoning an Order of Jesuits and booking myself in for an eight-day Ignation retreat.

Chapter 9

You will ask me next how to destroy this stark awareness of your own existence. For you are thinking that if it were destroyed all other difficulties would vanish too. And you would be right.

The Cloud of Unknowing

The journey to north Wales would have qualified as a small pilgrimage in itself. There was no direct line and I hunched frozen and wet on various train stations waiting for slow connections. The rain came lashing down, making the whole idea seem even more foolish and unattractive. I had started to have second thoughts about this course of action immediately after arranging it, partly because I hadn't the faintest idea of what to expect.

Within hours of leaving home I was cold and wet and nervous. It would probably take me a week to dry out. The place might be so austere and cold I'd die of pneumonia instead of cancer. I was always looking for other things to die of, wondering what they would put on the death certificate. Would I still be a cancer statistic if I drowned at sea during one of my unequal struggles with a windsurfer? I was doing quite well as a statistic. No doubt Issels had me on record somewhere, certainly Contreras had, and I'd now started popping up all over the place. Someone had sent me an article from a magazine published in the antipodes which referred to a woman with breast cancer who was reputed to have pulled off some amazing self-cure using a combination of meditation and magic. I was just on the point of finding out more about this fascinating phenomenon when I realized it was supposed to be about me ...

It was getting dark as I arrived, but the rain was just a bit less punishing as I waited limply at the station according to instructions. I tried to get myself into gear, to prepare myself in some way for the week ahead, but I couldn't imagine what one did in these circumstances. No doubt if you were a monk or a nun there would be some kind of form or ritual, unknown to me, that preceded retreats, which made me wonder – not for the first time – why, as a layman, I thought I qualified for this sort of exercise. A sharp start of panic accompanied the thought that I might be expected to know what I was looking for, that someone might ask me why I was there, a question I couldn't really answer. Certainly an acquaintance of mine had claimed her breast cancer had healed as a direct result of sorting herself out spiritually, but I was far too cynical or realistic to imagine that such a thing would happen to me. It would certainly sound a rather inappropriate motivation and one I would never have owned up to, even if it were true.

A small car rattled into the station yard, disgorging an apologetic figure who threw my bags into the back, bundled me into the passenger seat and hurled the door shut, all in what seemed like a single movement. He was back in his seat in a flash, hardly a spot of rain on him.

'If we hurry we'll get back in time for supper. I've asked them to save something for us.'

Obviously a prolonged fast was not part of the schedule.

The priest told me his name and said it was he who would 'guide' my retreat. He would come along to my room later and explain what that meant, meantime to tell him a bit about myself.

What bit, I wondered, would he like to hear? The 'wonderful wife and mother, coping bravely against impossible odds' bit, the 'I've tried every holistic therapy known to man and decided to bail out into the arms of God' bit, the 'I haven't the faintest idea what to do next and I'm in the most terrible muddle' bit. I pulled out one image of myself after another and had a look at each one before deciding that wasn't quite the impression I wanted to make and putting it away again. But why was I trying to impress him anyway? Why did I want to say what I thought would

145

please him most? That wasn't why I had come, to be a big hit with a Jesuit priest.

I sat hypnotized by the windscreen washers and the sibilation of the rain and wished I could, just for once, know who I was behind all these performances. I didn't want to parade a stylized version of myself, I wanted to express who I was behind all that and didn't know how to. Germany and subsequent events had opened me up to the idea that 'I' wasn't my performance or my role or my fear or my cancer or whatever, so now I knew who 'I' wasn't, but I still didn't know who I was. Funny that this should have been so quickly exposed by this man. Was it because he was a priest? Almost certainly.

I peered through the rain into the falling dusk as if I might get some inspiration from so unpromising a source. Hoping perhaps that an image of what I wanted to say would slowly develop before me, like a polaroid picture. With a lot of throat-clearing and croaking I informed him that I had a husband, three children and a tumour in my breast. It seemed to satisfy him, but I was fascinated at how ridiculous it sounded to me.

I wonder if everyone has the same reaction on being received into St Beuno's as Gerald Manley Hopkins had when he entered there as a young Jesuit student? He spoke of the warmth and kindness extended to him, 'deserving no such thing'. I certainly felt the same, but then I doubt if very much has changed from that day to this. Except, if Hopkins' letter to his father about the heating is to be believed, I think it's a bit warmer now. It didn't take me a week to dry out – I had a radiator bravely taking on the challenge of a twelve foot ceiling and about twenty square feet of window, and a tiny little electric fire. It was very warm and welcoming.

I grew to love the room. It had the proportions of a miniature cathedral with internal stone mullions which were quite beautiful. The door was immense and opened on to the main corridor, which ran the whole of the length of one side of the building. Any excursions to the bathroom required negotiating the full length of this corridor which, at night, was no mean feat, since I could never remember where the light switches were. There was quite a bit of furniture dotted around, chairs, bookcases, and an almost life-size statue of the Virgin Mary. In an attempt not to crash into any of these I used to creep through the inky blackness with my hands stretched out in front of me like someone playing Blind Man's Buff. What with that, and my long white nightie, I would have made a convincing ghostly apparition, but fortunately I never met anyone else on my nightly travels.

However, I was not alone. St Bueno's was very busy, full to capacity with a large group of men and women, all of whom were heavily and practically committed to the spiritual life. There were monks and nuns and fathers and priests and mother superiors and missionaries, all in their last week of a three-month training period that they had spent together. This exercise had begun with a full, thirty-day Ignation retreat. An achievement so prodigious, my own eight-day version started to look quite wimpish. As things turned out I barely survived the week – a month would have seen the end of me.

Although I had not really known what to expect, I had a pretty good idea of what I was not expecting. I didn't imagine, for example, that I would get to be so angry that I could barely be civil to my retreat leader, nor had I reckoned with the endless, barren hours of despair. But what came as the biggest shock of all was that nobody seemed to care. When I told my tale to my retreat leader later that night he didn't react to it at all. Any more than he had in the car. Even when I politely fleshed out the details for him, so he could see that my emotional and spiritual needs were for real, more urgent and pressing than most people's, he still didn't seem to understand. I thought perhaps he was a bit dim, after all it wasn't fair to assume all incumbents enjoy a dazzling intellect. I planned to put it all more clearly in the morning. He explained that he would visit me twice a day for between fifteen minutes and half an hour, morning and evening. During this time he would give me a spiritual exercise of some sort, a meditation, a contemplation, a specific text to study. As a general rule retreatants were not expected to talk, except to their retreat leader, so at mealtimes I should sit on the table specially reserved for people maintaining silence. Television and novels and so on were, quite reasonably,

147

discouraged, but going out for walks was considered a good idea.

He returned after breakfast the next day and gave me my exercise. I revamped my tragedienne, 'I might be dying' number, and he said softly, 'We're all dying.'

Now this was not news to me, it was something I had said many times to myself, and even to other people, in an attempt to keep things in perspective, but nobody had ever said it to me before. Nobody had ever shown a detached lack of interest in my suffering, made me feel that it wasn't particularly important, almost brushed the details aside. He acknowledged it of course, he accepted that I was suffering, and that as a result I was wrestling with fears and anxieties, but saw this as part of the human condition. Part of the way things are. Nobody could corner the market. Suffering is suffering is suffering. No particular suffering is more special, or more worthy of attention than any other. My having cancer was not significant, although how I felt about having it – that might be significant, he was interesed in that.

For the first time in four years I dropped the idea of the cancer being important. I didn't have to play any of the roles associated with it: the wounded healer, the impeccable warrior, the pathetic specimen. The man sitting opposite me was not interested in any of this. I did not have to have cancer in order to be driven on in the quest for peace. Anyone could sit here cracking under what Ainslie would have described as 'the anxiety of being alive' without justifying their right to do so on the basis of being sick. Or even mortally sick.

For a brief period I revelled in the sense of freedom that this brought me, but it didn't last long. The 'who am I question' was even more difficult to answer if I didn't have the cancer to play around with. Hour by hour, day by day every last refuge was stripped away from me. I grew angrier and more desperate than ever. My retreat leader remained impassive. I railed and wept and complained. He came and went. Each time I struggled desperately to involve him, trying frantically to externalize my pain, make him do something about it, or at least show me what to do, but every encounter was the same: another exercise that pointed me back to myself, back to God. I was thoroughly fed up with my retreat leader by this time, but I was reserving the heavy guns for God himself.

When I finally gave in to the idea that there was only Him and me in this, I gave in also to the tidal wave of rage and resentment that I had been building up for the past four years but had never dared admit to. Not to believe in God at all would be terrible enough, but to believe in Him and feel furiously angry towards him seemed much worse. Appropriately enough my next exercise involved Job.

Job was a great comfort. I loved the continuous stream of his fury, disappointment, rancour and indignation. It was gratifying to note that he lived another one hundred and forty years after his crisis, so clearly God was not adverse to a good argument. Inspired by Job's fantastic peroration against his maker, I strode around the Welsh hills doing the same thing myself. My angry orations scattered the curious sheep in waves. It did cross my mind that I seemed to be making a habit of using – or should I say abusing? – good country walks with my violent outbursts, but I was beyond worrying about this or controlling it. Anyway, I guess the local residents had seen it all before. Certainly one old man who blocked my path one afternoon was well versed in the routines.

'Eight day, or thirty day?' he enquired, referring to the length of my retreat. 'Route one or route three?'

This was a reference to the length of my walk. Some thoughtful soul had kindly prepared and photocopied some guide maps for the use of newcomers to the area. Obviously this old man knew every inch of every route. He was standing at a crucial junction ready to direct me appropriately. Most kind. I'd been feeling a distinct lack of this sort of authoritarian directing in recent times, and, despite the maps, I had managed to get lost once or twice. (Of course I blamed God for this as well.)

By the middle of the week I was in tatters and fully expecting my retreat leader to suggest we called it a day. As is my wont under stress I cried almost continuously. This grew to be a bit of a problem because I looked so puffy-eyed and flushed I knew that anyone who set eyes on me would know I was in a state of collapse. I felt a bit self-conscious about this,

149

surrounded as I was by all these 'holy' people – professional retreatants you might say. Survivors of the thirty-day marathon yet. But whenever I presented myself in the supper queue I sensed only their overwhelming empathy. Gradually, far from dreading exposure to them in the dining room, I almost looked forward to it, so strong were the feelings of love and support that they put out towards me. I felt this too when we met at daily mass.

Obviously, being a Jesuit house, this was a Catholic mass. The nearest I had come to a Catholic mass until then was trying to get into the line of fire of some holy water that was being sprayed over the crowds in a cathedral in Mexico. I had always thought Catholics to be rather exclusive and a bit stuffy about the presence of non-Catholics, and had not expected to be invited to join the group in its family service. I was therefore surprised and pleased to be welcomed into the little chapel. I learned a lot there.

Every service included a short homily, given by a member of the seminar group. Many of these men had parishes of their own and congregations of various sizes to look after, but one would never have been able to divine this just by looking at them. After all everyone was in mufti – pottering about in jeans and sweaters. It came as quite a shock to me to watch people I had last seen with their shirt tails hanging over a pair of checked trousers, sweep into the chapel draped in every imaginable piece of finery and gold thread. In the deep isolation of my retreat I pondered on the whole concept of carrying office and came out all the wiser for my contemplations.

After a few days it became clear that my retreat leader had no intention of giving up on me, although I think he wondered once or twice whether I would complete the course. It seemed an interminable time, that eight days. Oddly enough there was no comfort to be had from the 'four down, only another four to go' kind of reasoning. When the going was rough it was impossible to see a way out of it. There were no devices, or models, or styles or performances that could soften these sharp edges of self-knowledge. It was appalling. Was this what was meant by the long dark night

150

of the soul, the valley of the shadow of death? These were phrases never to be used lightly again.

I forgot all about my children, my husband, my patients, my cancer, my therapies. Stripped of all this I began to find out who I was.

There must have been a turning point during the week when I started to see the light at the end of the tunnel, but I don't recall that clearly. I only know that I was gradually restored, that a somewhat battered phoenix struggled feebly out of the ashes. I understood for the first time what Paul meant about God's strength being perfected in our weakness. I had come through.

On the last evening of my stay I left the retreatants' table and joined all the others. They were ebullient with warmth towards me, running forth and back to fetch me food and drinks, recalling incidents that had taken place during the week.

'We felt sorry for you, you were obviously having such a hard struggle. It can be pretty terrible can't it!'

I hadn't expected this. Could it be 'pretty terrible' for them too? I mean, I thought they were experts at this sort of thing.

'My dear, it's like that for everyone. We knew what you were going through because we've all been through it ourselves. The funny thing is that it doesn't seem to get any easier however many times you do it. Despair is a necessary part of any retreat.'

This was a revelation to me. We talked on and on. They shared as much as they could of their own experiences with me.

One of the priests had been so miserable he said he used to get up at night and wander around the building weeping. He was such a tough-looking, craggy-faced man it was difficult to imagine such a thing, but everyone insisted they had all felt the same. We sat around laughing and joking, making the most of the short time that was left, knowing that the chances of ever meeting again in this way were slim indeed. They were about to depart to their various seminaries, mission posts, hospitals and convents, all bearing different degrees of responsibility and authority. Strengthened by all

151

that they had learned and experienced during their three months, but taking with them also a better knowledge of their weaknesses and inadequacies.

I felt immeasurably better for having faced my weaknesses, for having peered into the void and stood before my fears. Of course I would be frightened again, I hadn't seen the last of that, but something about me had changed. I had truly let go. I knew now for sure that underneath are the Everlasting Arms.

Towards the end of the evening I decided to ring David and arrange for him to meet me from the train. I was very excited about talking to him and collected some change for the pay-phone. I then experienced the weirdest of all witnesses to the depth of the withdrawal I had made during the last week. I couldn't remember my own telephone number. I tried every trick in the book – not thinking about it for a while, and then sort of mentally sneaking upon myself – but nothing was any good. The really ridiculous part was the fact that we had an ex-directory number so I couldn't find out from directory enquiries. In the end I had to abandon the whole idea and ring David at work the following day. If he was surprised at the way I had wiped out of my mind what might have been considered as fairly essential data, he didn't show it.

Taking advantage of the cloud of euphoria that surrounded me, just before leaving I discussed the possibility of returning to do the full thirty-day retreat. In a diary I kept of the events of that week I wrote, 'I have raised this question of the thirty-day retreat with several people, mainly because I am actually terrified at the prospect, I think, and would change my mind if I hadn't committed myself all round.'

Very wisely my retreat leader said they would consider me for this, but left the matter unresolved and open-ended. When I do return it will be out of choice, not obligation. Mind you, I shall have to consider this carefully. Who knows what I shall have forgotten about myself after a month?

There was a big change in me on my return home, apparent to everyone who saw me. The depression had gone, I felt altogether steadier and brighter. I decided on a regime for myself that I thought best suited my needs and quietly got on with it. I went to see Dr Howard who pronounced my situation unchanged, and very cautiously I started to pick up the threads of my life again.

I was very much looking forward to another seminar at the Cancer Help Centre, this time to be given by Hans Moolenburg, a Dutch physician. I already knew Hans slightly since he had visited the Centre before and had worked closely with Alec Forbes in the past. The board of directors of the Centre were well aware of how much we could learn from this man, and a weekend had been arranged during which he was to give a seminar at the Centre and spend time discussing potential developments.

Hans is the original Gentle Giant.

It was he who first coined the phrase 'the gentle method' as a way of describing his approach to cancer, and for years we have all drawn extensively on his wide knowledge and experience.

I was deputed to meet him at the airport, and did so willingly. For one thing he is an easy person to meet in a crowded place for the simple reason that he is about a foot taller than anyone else. For another he is one of the nicest people I know. Like many very tall men he is also quite slim, but he gives an overall impression of strength. He has what can only be described as a boyish grin, and this gives him an almost ingenuous look at times, but this is deceptive, he is both wise and wily. He needs to be. Like most doctors who do not toe the party line he attracts a lot of attention in his native Holland – not all of it desirable. Fortunately this has not caused him to become angry or bitter. Quite the contrary, he revels in the funny side of the occasional confrontations he has with the authorities and recounts these with a refreshing, acerbic wit. He has a laugh like a fog horn and it was a pleasure to see him again.

He gave his usual stylish dissertation at the Centre. Offering a gathering of concerned and interested doctors an opportunity to broaden their horizons in relation to the treatment and management of cancer patients. He has an eclectic overview of medicine that is postively dazzling to the conventionally trained doctor who has never expanded his

153

thinking beyond the patient's skin. It must have been extraordinary for some of them to hear Hans moving smoothly from the concept of a 'cancer personality' developing in the mind, to ways in which this might encourage neoplasmic changes in the body, and what to do about both. I find him a stimulating and exciting person to be with, and the rest of the weekend produced some lively discussions between us all.

During the break for tea he switched from the general to the particular and asked me how I was getting on personally. Not an easy question to answer because, although I felt good in my head and my heart, my lumpy breast suggested that things were far from good physically.

'What about Iscador?' he asked. 'Do you not take Iscador also?'

I knew that Iscador was the brain-child of Rudolph Steiner who had some very enlightened and attractive views on the subject of health and disease. Faithful to the homoeopathic principle of 'like cures like', he had developed a nostrum for cancer based on mistletoe which he saw as behaving in a way very similar to the disease: a parasite that thrived at the expense of its host. Iscador is an extract of mistletoe, mixed with various different substances according to the type of cancer it is intended to treat, and administered in various ways, but usually by subcutaneous injection. I had often given some thought to pursuing this treatment, but until Hans' suggestion had not mobilized myself into doing so. This was mainly because I knew I would need the services of an anthroposophical doctor which would mean another consultation. I wasn't sure I could face grinding my way through my past history yet again, and having to find a rational slot for yet one more treatment in the colourful patchwork of my existing therapies. Several things inspired me to carry on in this direction: Hans' evident enthusiasm, my own positive feelings about it, and the fact that, after weeks of inner discussions about whether to do it or not, I discovered that I could pronounce 'anthroposophical' without stuttering or clenching my teeth. This struck me as a good omen so I made an appointment.

I should have known it would all go very smoothly because I had felt so good about it from the beginning. The doctor knew enough about me already to make the case-taking quite quick and painless, and he was optimistic about the use of Iscador for me.

'In your case I think the prognosis is good. You are already eating properly and you have the right mental outlook. I'll write to your doctor and tell him what I've suggested you do.'

His suggestions were that I should have regular, repeated courses of injections, that I should administer these injections myself, and that they should be given directly into the breast itself. The aspect of this that shocked me the most was that I didn't mind. If anyone had suggested years before that I should do anything as gross and aggressive as injecting a foreign substance bang into the area around my miscreant cells I would never have accepted it. To my great surprise I was quite ready to do this and for some time I mused over the changes that had taken place in my attitudes over the years.

I thought about the discussion with the American psychotherapist who had said I was a different person now. I listened again to the tape of our conversation and heard myself saying that this tumour wasn't necessary to me. Whereas at first cancer had been important, it was now redundant. It was time for it to go. No wonder I felt quite cheerful about encouraging it on its way in so un-compromising a fashion. I actually enjoyed giving myself these injections and accompanied them with some mighty powerful visualizations and verbal instructions.

There was just one slight problem. Each injection raised a firm round lump in my breast which took several days to disperse. Each shot followed on so quickly from the other, there was never enough time for one lump to go before another took its place. Sometimes, by the end of two weeks there were lots of lumps making themselves felt in different parts of my breast. The anthroposophical doctor assured me that this was normal and they would all disappear in time, so this wasn't a problem for me. I realized on the other hand that they would present something of a problem for Dr Howard. It didn't seem fair, in view of his meticulous efforts to measure my progress, to present him with a breast that felt

155

like a bag full of marbles. This meant I had to time my visits to him to coincide with the week in between courses of Iscador when my tissues returned to their normal state. Even so, I felt obliged to tell him about my latest foray into self-medication. His response was not encouraging. He indulged in a slightly quizzical expression, sighed, and started to say, 'In my experience ...'

It was obvious what was coming and I could do without it. Rather rudely I interrupted him, 'Please don't say anything. Well, not unless it's something positive and encouraging anyway.'

He didn't say anything.

Increasingly I made myself look at my changing attitudes, both to having a tumour and what to do about it. I tried to steer clear of the idea that there was any right or wrong in this, a better or a best way of responding. The fact was I responded to my situation according to my needs. In the early days of my cancer crisis my needs had been for holistic help and, ironically, since cancer was my way into getting this help, there was a sense in which I needed the cancer as well. But all the intervening years of therapy, meditation and counselling had not been in vain: those needs had been met, I didn't need to have a tumour any longer. I had no doubt at all that I now had other needs, but I felt capable of reaching out into areas that would fulfil them without the justification of a life-threatening disease. Following through the tangents of my thinking in this way also enabled me to cope with having changed my mind. I no longer felt that this was some kind of misdemeanour that required either apology or absolution. I felt perfectly at ease with the idea that these changes were part of an organic growth that was taking place in me and, as such, were both inevitable and desirable. In this comfortable frame of mind I forced myself to examine my dogmatic attitude to radiotherapy treatment.

For months now I had been returning regularly to see Dr Howard. Our meetings were blessed with a certain predictability: he always booked a session for me on the radiotherapy machine in the belief that I would surely need it, and I always managed to wriggle out of it on the basis of his exhaustive examination and assiduous measuring. He was prepared to go along with this, cancelling my slot on the treatment list with a tolerant good grace, but I was never in any doubt that he was a reluctant party to my refusing treatment, and was always hoping that I would change my mind. In my new, relaxed state of mind I looked more closely at my persistent refusal. It seemed to me that I was doggedly holding on to a rather outworn view of my situation. The argument that aggressive, interventionist therapy would loosen my grip on my personal progress just didn't make sense any more. I didn't need to have this lump – indeed, I was very keen to get rid of it. If Dr Howard thought he could vaporize it with a burst or three of his Star Wars gun, then why on earth didn't I let him?

There seemed to be no justification whatsoever for my stubborn resistance, except perhaps my pride. I was a bit worried about this because there was no doubt that pride was a factor that was at work here. In fairness I did then, and do now, believe that radiotherapy, in common with many other current cancer therapies, will soon be overtaken by new techniques. That one day we shall wander around radio-therapy departments in much the same way as we visit museums, wondering at the monstrous apparatus and paraphernalia that was once thought so efficacious. But even if that is so, that these techniques will take their place alongside leeches and suchlike, this does not mean that they do not have their place in the unfolding of wisdom and understanding. Surely any right-minded person would avail themselves of the best that is currently on offer, not dream about a Utopia yet to come? And if they didn't, what was stopping them? Pride maybe. I decided to let this go, along with quite a few of my other illusions about myself. I would give Dr Howard the surprise of his life and let him loose his high-technology wizardry on to my carefully measured lumps.

Although my encounters with Dr Howard were a quantum improvement on any previous medical consult-ations I had participated in, I still found it challenging to present myself to the hospital, to take my place in a system that served sick people, and generally play the role of patient. It was impossible not to feel terribly nervous, since lurking at the back of my mind was the possibility that something dreadful might have happened that I hadn't noticed, and then I would suddenly find myself out of my depth, impotent, back on the road to being a victim again. I never found it easy. I certainly didn't look for opportunities to go when I didn't have to, so Dr Howard might well have been surprised when I arranged an early appointment. I decided not to tell David. If I needed him to hold my hand then I wasn't as strong as I needed to be for what I had in mind. On the way up in the train I tested my reactions to the possibility that this time my place on the machine would not be cancelled. This time I might have to face the thick lead door closing tightly behind me. (Some I had seen had a skull and cross-bones stencilled on the outside, not something likely to inspire confidence in any but the most intrepid.) Would I then be left alone, vulnerable and exposed, while my attendants scuttled off behind the safety of lead aprons and high screens? Would I be able to feel strong and confident under such conditions? Yes I would. My life was wonderful and precious to me, I would put all my will and positivity into this, I would simply *make* it work.

Dr Howard had, not unnaturally, assumed a change for the worst. I assured him that as far as I knew nothing had happened physically, but I felt more relaxed now about the radiotherapy, and thought I ought to give him the benefit of a consultation that did not have to carry the weight of my bias. I think he was quite surprised.

'Well, let's have a look and see what's going on.'

We went smoothly through our usual routine. He looked and felt and measured. He went to his desk and scrutinized his notes and drawings. He came back and measured me again. He went back to his desk, fiddled about with his pencil, gazed into the middle distance, let out a long sigh and earned for himself the Gentle Giant award.

'I don't think I ought to give you radiotherapy treatment at the moment. The fact is that you appear to be in control of whatever is going on here. I can't pretend to understand this, but I do know that it would be madness to interfere with what appears to be a stable situation.'

I wonder sometimes if he was ever tempted to go ahead

anyway, thereby sucking me into his world, a world he understood so well, where he was unquestionably in charge, in control. That would surely have been so much easier for him than continuing to operate in this grey twilight zone with me. The fact that he opted to do so, that he was big enough to set aside his chosen theories and continue to do his best to support me along the way he knew I preferred, that increased my faith in him even more. He enjoyed telling his secretary that now I had admitted to a change of heart he had decided to withhold his wares. We all laughed about it, I made another appointment for three months' time, and within an hour I was back on the train.

David just didn't know what to make of it all. He had a bit of catching up to do in my mental processes and was understandably confused, but of course he grasped at once the significance of the day's events.

'If you weren't fighting him over the treatment and he said you didn't need it, surely you must see how wonderful that is.'

Of course I did, but it was good to hear him say it. Try as I might I couldn't effect as detached a calm as I would have liked. I doubt if I shall ever be that cool, but I am slowly moving towards a more detached view of what is happening to me. I think I dare claim to have exercised some control over what Eliot refers to as 'undisciplined squads of emotions'. But with my track record maybe I shouldn't talk too soon . . .

Chapter 10

We shall not cease from exploration
And the end of all our exploring
Will be to arrive where we started
And know the place for the first time.
                                                    T.S. Eliot

One of my favourite Snoopy cartoons shows a picture of him writing a book. He is typing away furiously, sheets of paper flying out of the machine and wobbling into loose piles around him. Then with a nervous and unconvincing grimace he announces that he will shortly be pulling all this lot together. I know how he feels. This is the hard part. It is all the harder for me because I have deliberately avoided writing a prescriptive book, and even rounding off with a conclusion invites the temptation to quantify and qualify and make judgements about the events of the last six years. I am very reluctant to do this because what was right for me may not be right for anyone else. Anyway, one has to ask in what sense any of this has been 'right' even for me. Has any healing taken place, and if so, healing of what?

On the physical level it's hard to say what has happened, or what is going on now. Mercifully everything seems very static and quiet at the moment, but technically I still have a tumour in my breast, and I'd never get a job as a topless waitress. (I am not comforted by the retort one of my friends made in response to this observation – 'But Penny, you don't *want* a job as a topless waitress!' – because I'm the sort of person who would like to have the offer and then turn it down.) So, from the pathological perspective it is far from clear what, if anything, I have achieved. Nevertheless I have managed to duck – or at the very least postpone – some of the heavier, more destructive cancer treatments and that can only be good. The lifestyle that I have adopted gives me more energy than I ever had before I was ill and this enables me to live a much fuller life, which I consider to be a great bonus. I continue to care very much about what happens to my physical body and I have all sorts of hopes and expectations with regard to my full recovery, but I now feel able to pursue such therapies as I feel will be a means to this end without the histrionic attachment to survival that I once had.

The most noticeable change that has taken place in me over the past few years has been to do with an increased detachment on my part. Sometimes, but of course not all the time, I am able to be my own wise observer. From this position it is possible to contemplate with reasonable equanimity the hope of my full physical recovery and at the same time accept the possibility that I shall not conquer this disease. Such peace and stability as I have acquired comes from being able to cope with either outcome: success or failure, life or death.

There was a time when I thought that simultaneously maintaining two opposites was a form of madness. I had been taught to believe that you simply couldn't do this: either I am cured of cancer and going to live a long time, or I am not, and might die pretty soon. I used to believe that one of these statements about my position had to be the reality and the other an illusion, I no longer believe this to be so.

Then what is the difference between illusion and reality? Possibly there is none. For me anyway, reality is whichever illusion I currently feel happy with. 'To be or not to be' is no longer the question. The question is how to be both.

Grappling with this paradox is no longer the frustrating struggle that it was. This is because of what has been happening to me at a non-physical level. Although my initial motivation when I started meditating and using visualization techniques was to enhance my capacity to heal myself physically, as I continued with these methods I found that I was pursuing them for different reasons. Gradually I found myself less and less attracted to images of small white sharks (leukocytes) eating up a cauliflower (the tumour).

161

Perhaps I wouldn't have a lump now if I had concentrated more on this side of things, but what really interested me was the potential for psychological and spiritual growth that seemed to open up when I spent at least some part of the day in a different reality. By disengaging briefly from the world of action and existing for a while without doing anything, just being, I found myself acquiring some much needed strength and tranquility. The change that this brought about in the quality of my life was so great that the goal of getting rid of cancer cells receded a bit.

Much the same thing happened with counselling. Although it was hard to see how counselling would get rid of tumours, I had maintained from the very beginning that my emotional muddle was part of my sickness, so obviously untangling the Gordian knot of my relationships had to be part of the cure. Incidentally, the Gordian was never untied: Alexander the Great took the easy way out and axed it open. But I was never tempted to take any short-cuts in this area, it was so fascinating and enthralling I couldn't get enough of it. Increasingly I found that cancer featured less and less in the encounters I had with various facilitators and counsellors, because everything else was so much more interesting. It was far more important to me that I should do something about my 'unfinished business' than come up with a clean bill of health.

Healing of a non-physical kind has certainly taken place. From the space that I occupy at the moment I can say unequivocally that this is the healing I needed, the healing I sought, and that it is sufficient for me. But, even as I write, I know perfectly well that if I woke up tomorrow with enlarged glands, or another lump, I should soon be singing another song. And why not? I have learned to allow myself to respond to challenges in whatever way feels right at the time. My feelings about my present situation are quite different from those that prevailed when I was first ill. I can live with that: I can live with the idea that they might change again. All that matters is to be able to cope with the way I'm feeling now.

Through knowing myself and accepting myself a little better I find it easier to live for now. To be fully in this moment. While I was a seething mass of guilts and fears I was for ever plotting and planning ways to improve everything – myself, my status, my performance. I didn't want to live for the present moment because it was always tangled up with my past failures and never as good as the mythical futures I was dreaming up. The healing that I know has taken place lies in this: that the present is all right with me. I have quite a complicated web of future projections: some short-term, some long-term, some private, some public. Only one thing has changed: I now find I am able to plan my future without depending on having it.

Of course this doesn't mean that I never project myself into the future, I do it all the time. Indeed I think that our capacity to visualize new pleasures and successes and delights for ourselves is very healthy. If all we listen to is the poor prognosis from the hospital and the head-shaking pity of our friends, then we run a very serious risk of becoming a self-fulfilling prophecy and dying because that's what society expects us to do. It is necessary for us to give ourselves another scenario to work with, one that requires us to be alive. This then becomes the antidote to the heavy death spell that is cast by the cancer diagnosis.

People have different ways of doing this. Parents often attach themselves to the idea of living to see a daughter married or a grandchild born. I am currently watching with interest the sprightly progress of a man so angry about something his consultant once said to him he is resolute in his plan to outlive the man as a kind of revenge. These are only other versions of the goals I used to set myself – cycling in France, windsurfing and so on. It is, however, quite important to keep revising one's objectives. It's no good dropping dead the minute you achieve something just because there's nothing else to live for.

However I do not expect myself to maintain this guru-like strength and wisdom for long periods of time. There are days when I can't do it at all and find myself reaching out in search of the comforting reassurance that I am not dying. I have various ways of coping with these times. One well-tested, time-honoured technique is to turn to David and say I feel terrible and does he think I'm going to be all right. This is his cue to come up with the structural engineer's view of cancer control, and as long as it's positive it will do fine. The point is that there are times when the burden feels too heavy and one turns to others to lend a hand. Sometimes I experience periods of such weakness that I would willingly withdraw every strong-willed statement I've ever made, and at such times the need for outside support and encouragement becomes very great. However, I have learned that there is never sufficient reassurance to cover the really big existential fears, and if I continue to feel the need for external props and supports of this sort, then it's time to look inwards and draw on my own resources.

Thus it is that on a good day I can sit loose to the idea of living or dying, enjoying fully just my being here, now. At other times my fears and anxieties come seeping through like a persistent, insidious rising damp, but I'm more in touch with these feelings now and have developed mechanisms for dealing with them. Some of these mechanisms concern my inner being, but some of them are very much to do with my day-to-day life. Setting and achieving even small goals does wonders for the morale. I have just bicycled fifty-six miles from London to Brighton. Hardly a recommended cancer cure, but wondrous good for the ego.

Like most people I am hardly ever creative. Crippled by the protestant work ethic I somehow manage to turn everything I do into being productive or useful or significant. It has required a deliberate act of discipline and will to join a class where I attempt to paint with watercolours. To my great delight I have not felt any compulsion to get to grips with the techniques. I still don't know what colours you have to mix in order to make green, but that feeling I get when breathless, with anticipation, I drop wet into wet is one of the greatest joys imaginable. More enjoyable still is the fact that those of my efforts that have been most admired have actually been controlled accidents. Rather like the events of the last few years, you might say.

Knowing how good it feels to do something like this I have tentatively returned to my violin playing. Unfortunately this has not been as socially acceptable. My musical career has been stunted somewhat by having a daughter who says, 'It's bad enough having a mother who plays the violin at all – I mean, at your age, that's really embarrassing – but to have a mother with orchestra hair, that's even worse.'

I am secretly much taken with the idea of having orchestra hair, but the warning signs are there. My children have tolerated a lot over the past few years. Now that I've given up on the idea that I shall ever be a Perfect Parent I feel it prudent to bend a little in their direction. I no longer insist on cosy musical evenings. Partly because of certain people's obvious reluctance to participate, but also because they were never that cosy. Rumour has it that I was just a shade bossy. I am learning to pursue one possibility and then, if necessary, let it go and try something else. For the first time in my life I don't feel some kind of a failure for doing this. The important thing has been to keep a balance between my physical, emotional, creative and spiritual needs and naturally this requires shifting around quite a bit.

It also requires that I should know what these needs are, and accept that they are uniquely mine.

What works for me may not work for you, but the general principle of listening to your own opinion of what your needs are, and having some say in choosing therapies that you feel will meet those needs – those things are important for us all. I have a good working relationship with literally dozens of different kinds of cancer treatments although I am currently involved with only a few. I keep myself informed about any new developments that I think might appeal to me, so there are plenty of new threads to weave into the tapestry if required. I might one day succumb to Dr Howard's matchless salesmanship; I have instructions on how to construct a healing pyramid to sleep under, which I have always rather fancied; I even found an old Chinese herbal remedy for cancer that was startingly imaginative, but since one of the key ingredients was a medium-sized baked toad I'd have to be pretty desperate to resort to that. I have lots of interesting possibilities open to me, but finding any one therapist who can advise me on them all is a bit unlikely.

When I was first ill I sought desperately, and in vain, for

someone who had been through the same experiences as me, so that I could follow them. I was sure that there must be someone out there who had trodden just the path I wanted to tread and left behind a nice, clear set of big, warm footprints. No sooner did I wake up to the fact that this was an unrealistic expectation than I found myself getting drawn into playing the part of Good King Wenceslas myself. Unfortunately, much as I understand this longing for leadership and clear guidance, I think it is only marginally helpful to adopt someone else's path.

We have to find our own way. This is difficult enough, but for anyone who is part of a culture that encourages the externalization of disease, it is harder still. The current pattern for dealing with disease is to take it along to an expert and give it to him. Choosing to be responsible for your own illness is not a comfortable position to be in. Less comfortable still, is the search to extract meaning from it.

The search for meaning in suffering is a popular sport amongst religious philosophers and is a bit easier from a library chair than a hospital waiting room, but it is a concept worth pursuing, anywhere. My nervous attempts at this brought me to the place where both the disease and how to cope with it became essentially my problem. I soon discovered that the only person who can carry the weight of this is God. My sisters were right about that, but this has to be Emanuel – God with us and within us – not a projected fantasy that looks like a cross between Neptune and Tolstoy glaring balefully down from a cloudy throne. If we are going to know the meaning of 'the Kingdom of Heaven is within you' we must embark on a more intimate relationship with God. Jesus said 'I am the Way' and this is the Way I have tried to find. 'I AM' is one of the earliest translations of the word for God.

It started long before I was ill, of course. As the child of a woman born and raised in the valleys of South Wales, one of my first conscious recollections was the sound of Cwm Rhondda rolling in eight-part harmony from the lips of the local male voice choir. Anyone who has felt the power of that shivering up through the soles of their feet, will never be indifferent to the idea of a trans-personal spiritual dimension.

166

And if having cancer is the way to 'Open now the crystal fountain whence the healing stream doth flow', then it's no bad thing to have.

Appendix

I have said several times already that it was never my intention to write a prescriptive book, and I do not intend this appendix to be seen as a therapeutic guide. My intention is merely to outline those aspects of the events of the past five years that I still consider to be important – the things that have stayed with me until now. For people wanting specific details and more information about ways of coping with cancer their best course of action would be to contact The Bristol Cancer Help Centre (see page 178).

With every bookstall shouting out the various merits of a plethora of self-help therapies, the problem for the cancer patient is no longer whether he can do anything for himself, but where on earth to start. (As time goes by, this evolves into the question of where to stop. But that comes later.)

The place to start is with something that *YOU* think is important. Before buying a single book, arranging any appointments with 'highly-recommended' practitioners, before allowing any decisions to be made on your behalf, settle down and think about what is happening to you and how you want to see the problem solved. However impotent your surroundings may make you feel, nobody can stop you doing this. Allow yourself the luxury of exploiting your own reactions and responses to your crisis.

Talking with patients at The Bristol Cancer Help Centre has revealed to me that many people have their own ideas about what needs healing. These are usually rather broader based than the doctor's perspective. I remember well a man who proclaimed confidently,

'I reckon I know why I'm ill. Most of my life I've been a vegetarian, a bit of a health-nut really, then I got this job on the oil-rig – to make a bit more money – and I ate more meat in three months than I had in ten years. Got cancer of the colon didn't I? Well, stands to reason doesn't it?'

It didn't apparently stand to the reason of his consultant, who dismissed ideas about nutrition having anything to do with anything as the usual load of old nonsense he'd come to expect from patients who didn't know any better. I think to ask the question about who is right or wrong in this situation is to miss the point. It doesn't matter very much. What matters is that this patient's strong ideas about why he was ill moved him towards taking positive and specific action about getting better. His view of his situation was so clear and convincing to him even his consultant's cynicism couldn't dent it. However he felt the consultant had a point or two to make: he underwent surgery and then came to Bristol for advice about diet. For him, nutrition was the first and most important part of his self-help plan.

Another woman who came was obsessed with the thought that her cancer was a punishment for something she had done. She didn't think *ANYTHING* would help her: any treatment was a waste of time. She felt so guilty she wasn't surprised she had cancer and knew she would die because she thought she deserved to. Improved nutrition is not the most promising way forward for such a person. She is telling us what she needs – she needs counselling first and foremost. The point is, she knew what she needed.

Maybe you know what you need. Allow yourself to think about it and start there. You may not be able to express any of these thoughts to anybody else, but that doesn't matter right away. While you are being bombarded from all sides with advice based on everyone else's opinions of what is happening and what should be done, take some time to ask yourself if you agree with them or not. If you do agree then is this because you are too frightened to do anything else, or is it that you really feel the same? If your feelings about what should be done line up perfectly with those of the people around you then you will be able to pursue whatever therapy they suggest with heart and with enthusiasm. No problems there. If, on the other hand, you have the feeling that not everything matches up so nicely, then try to establish in your own mind which of your needs are not being met. Then, like the chap from the oil-rig, you may choose to accept the therapy on offer to you, but at the same time quietly determine to seek healing in other areas as well.

Start with those thoughts and feelings about your situation that are important to you – even if they don't matter to anybody else. In my case I believed that I was sick in my mind and spirit as well as in my body. Had I submitted to all the physical therapy in the world, it would still not have been enough. In my head I held on to the idea that I needed help on mental and spiritual levels as well, consequently concentrating on the physical was just not enough. I had a tendency at that time (which continues to this day) to consider my emotional problems my biggest challenge, and so I would be bound to say that counselling in its various forms rates very high with me.

Counselling

Counselling is not what it says it is. The word 'counsel' means to advise or give suggestions. This is what we get from lawyers or beauticians, it is not what we should be getting from the kind of counsellors I am referring to. Anyway, who wants it? I have never been short of people flooding me with their advice and suggestions, I don't need to pay someone else to do it as well. What I have been short of is help with the unravelling of my own convoluted thinking. What is it that I really think? Against the background noise of everyone else's clatter it is sometimes hard to listen to what we have to say to ourselves. A good counsellor will assist you in establishing your own counsel.

Who to go to?

The most unexpected people can turn out to be good counsellors, it isn't always necessary to go to professionals. In any assessment of my progress I would want to give my husband an enormous amount of credit for the help he gave me. However in between the sessions we have had together we have also availed ourselves, both singly and as a couple, of the skills of professionals. We have even, (more rarely,) joined in group work. Although untrained willing friends and relatives can be wonderful listeners, at the end of the day I think counselling is skilled and demanding work that is best undertaken by a professional.

I am presently watching with awe as a friend of mine staggers through his second year of a full Jungian analysis. This seems to involve at least three weekly sessions of considerable duration with his analyst, and I do sometimes wonder if there is enough time left in between visits for anything to happen in his life that would be worth analysing. All this means, of course, is that I am not attracted to this course of action myself, but it is a most fruitful course of action for some.

For a while I saw a counsellor fairly regularly. Now I just make an appointment when I feel the need. What is this need? It is the need to have someone to be there, listening, while I pursue new possibilities; bounce new ideas around; express things I cannot say to anyone too close to me. Also, from time to time I need someone to reflect back to me what I already know but cannot see clearly. In this sense a counsellor acts like a mirror. At other times I feel the need for a more detached observer than I can be for myself. This is like having someone sitting at the back of the hall at orchestra rehearsal. He is going to hear what the cellos are up to much better than the tympanist ever will, or even the conductor himself.

I wouldn't last ten minutes with a counsellor who tried to conduct for me the way I wish to play my life, but I am grateful for occasional feed-back about my over-all progress in putting the notes in the right order.

Anyone who feels that they have a crisis with an emotional component would do well to seek counselling. Not everyone flings themselves into a full-blown existential crisis at the mere sound of the word cancer, but most people who ever have the disease will know that it means more to them than bodily suffering. Over the years physical medicine has tragically divorced itself from psychological and spiritual healing, so don't be too surprised if all your needs can't be met in hospital.

Meditation, Relaxation and Visualization

This is a wonderfully exciting field, full of all sorts of fantastic possibilities. It is also full of all sorts of peculiar people, not all of whom will be at a stage where they will be able to help you. So ask around, read a few books, feel your way in gently, don't be afraid to have a go by yourself. Although my early, untutored efforts may sound a bit ridiculous – eyes squinting, foot braced against the door – the strange thing is that I recall some of those times as positive peaks of experience.

I was attracted to these techniques because I had unknowingly been flirting around with them most of my life. As a child I could readily and easily float up to the top right hand corner of my bedroom and watch myself and my sister in the beds below. I thought everybody did this to refresh themselves at the end of the day. I didn't know it was 'an out of body experience' and possibly a bit unusual. I only knew it felt terrific. If the going got really rough: geography homework returned as unmarkable yet again; dropped from the cricket team; history book irretrievably lost; nagging tooth-ache, I always knew I could glide into a place where none of these things mattered, where everything was well. I needed no persuading later in my life that I could retreat in my mind to places where cancer couldn't get me either.

Most of us have some vague, unformed belief that the mind is important, that it can be used to heal or hurt, but we don't know how to utilise it as part of our healing process. Unfortunately it is not enough to make all sorts of promises to oneself about positive thinking. I have yet to meet the person going through a crisis who can manage more than a few seconds of cheerful positivity before being overwhelmed again by all the familiar fears. A woman came to Bristol a few months ago who told me about a talk she had had with a nursing sister just before her discharge from hospital. This well-meaning woman assured her patient,

'We find that people who are positive and optimistic are the ones who do best of all in your condition. So, off you go now, and, remember ... be positive and optimistic all the time.'

173

Two years later the poor woman was back again with a relapse.

'Obviously sister, I wasn't positive and optimistic enough.'

Put in this way we can see what a cruel, pointless bit of advice that turned out to be. In fact it just gave the patient something else to worry about. What it didn't give her was a way of achieving this prodigous feat. The regular daily practice of simple visualization techniques is a way of holding a picture in our minds of a different reality. Not the reality of diagnosis, tumours, pain and death, but a (different) picture of ourselves transcending these events, offering us an alternate reality, another picture for the mind to play with.

Deep relaxation and meditation open up the possibility of experiencing different states of consciousness. Making contact with our inner selves in this way enhances our intuitive understanding of our lives. Gradually there is a flow-on effect from the rather contrived, unnatural slots of time set aside for meditation, into the chaotic hurly-burly of the rest of our lives. Eventually we find ourselves making better decisions, feeling strong enough to live with the consequences of those decisions and generally opening up to fresh ways of experiencing the world.

Physical Therapy

I can't resist putting this last because of course it usually comes first. During the course of my investigations into the non-physical world there were times when I doubted if physical therapy had a place at all in what I wanted to do, but now I am convinced that it does.

Recently I had a most bizarre encounter with a young man who was a complete stranger to me but was clearly determined to tell me all his problems. Not wishing to encourage him too much I was keeping very quiet, but eventually, desperate to get a response from me, he asked, 'Don't you ever feel your life isn't worth living?'

I heard myself burst out instantly, 'No, I never feel like

174

that. My life is enormously precious to me.'

And as I said it I was overcome with the force of how true it was. My life *IS* enormously precious to me now in a way that I was never aware of before I was ill. My desperate wish to put the healing needs of my mind and spirit before those of my body had an element of despair in it. There was a sense in which I had given up on my physical life, my existence as a human being, and was backing the other side of myself, my soul, as the only viable alternative. Since then I have developed a more balanced view of myself and consequently I am daily more and more attracted to the idea of staying alive. To this end I pay a good deal more attention to my physical body.

In what way?

Well, first of all in very obvious and simple ways. I rest when I'm tired and I don't work so hard. I shudder to remember the regularity with which I ploughed on with my chores, head thumping, hands shaking, up half the night with the ironing, setting myself impossible standards: listening to what my mind had to say about working mothers having to prove something, not listening to my body complaining that I was asking too much. Now I acknowledge my body's needs and acquiesce to them when I can.

I also feed my body thoughtfully. (See Chapter 2)

I have never been able to make sense of the person who agonises over whether they have put 2 star or 4 star fuel in their car, but couldn't tell you the food value of what they themselves had for dinner.

I think it matters what you eat.

This is not the time to go into details about nutrition, but I think my physical body performs better on high quality food. I know this to be true from my own experience as a patient and I have observed it to be the case for many others from my perspective as their therapist. I am no longer absolutely neurotic about diets for cancer patients as I was once, but I am watchful of what I put into my body. If unpronounceable additives in packets and tins might cause tumours in rats if taken in large doses, then it doesn't make any sense to me to make my body battle with them in any dose at all. There are some things I can't avoid. I suspect the slow infiltration of nitrates into just about everything that grows can hardly be good for us, but what I can't change I don't worry about.

The irrepressible David is fast turning into an organic gardener to be reckoned with. Not bad going for someone whose erstwhile agricultural zenith was to know that 'the big ones are trees and the little ones are flowers.' Since every mouthful of food grown in this way represents hours of loving effort on his part I am convinced it can only have an enhancing, healing influence on me. The same is true of food carefully and lovingly prepared by friends. I'm sure what you eat is important, but how you feel when you eat it probably matters more. I remember my daughter Justine bursting in from school, sticky pink with the excitement of having cooked me a scone in the cooking corner.

'All the time I was making it I knew how good it was because it's *BROWN FLOUR*, which is just right for you, and I've made one each, but I want you to have mine as well!'

It also contained white sugar and butter and baking powder and salt, but if you are ever lucky enough to have someone prepare food for you with so much love I suggest you eat it and enjoy it. I certainly did. I can see her face now, flushed with the thrill of having done something wonderful and clever for me. I don't believe God plays dice with the universe or that such a gesture could be anything but good, but I know that man is gambling with his diet, and that he's gambling hard and fast.

It makes no sense to me to stress my digestive system with food containing a list of substances that sound like a first year chemistry kit.

By the same logic I don't smoke and I keep away from people who do.

These are things I can do for myself, but I also consult therapists and practitioners for their help in mending and repairing my physical body.

I have an instinctive empathy with homoeopathic medicine and feel I have been greatly strengthened by it. In addition to constitutional treatment I am currently munching my way through a long-term dose of something aimed

176

specifically at reducing the tumour in my breast. Meanwhile I am still a keen devotee of Iscador and continue faithfully with that regime.

Although I am still dodging the baked toad treatment I have a special place in my heart for Chinese medicine. From the very outset of my health problems I have been loved, supported and encouraged by Dr Evans, a brilliant acupuncturist who taught me a great deal during the years I worked with him. He now has the doubtful privilege of dealing with me as a patient, a challenge I know he has no wish to repeat with anyone else. I am sure he dreads the nosey way I read all my notes, my intense perusal of my pulse picture and my anxious analysis of his proposed plan of action; but worst of all must be the times when he has to cope with me arguing furiously about what I will and will not let him do. It must be hard to have your patient sit bolt upright on the couch, clutch both her feet and protest,

'If you're thinking of doing Kidney One* – forget it!'

My pain threshold gets lower and lower with every visit, while his tolerance level is improving no end. I really wonder sometimes what we would do without him because when David finds the strain of coping with me quite insupportable, then, (most appropriately,) his back gives out, and he too cripples into the waiting room for a dose of the beloved Evans-the-Pins.

Always there in the background is the hospital and Dr Howard. Strictly speaking he hasn't yet actually given me any treatment, but that's a technicality. For the past two years I have had access to a doctor who I respect and trust which has been healing in itself. I feel comforted by the thought that the mighty arsenal of conventional cancer weapons is available to me, if ever the need for additional deterrents arises. But if it came to that I might even give in gracefully to Kidney One.

There is a tendency to get a bit over-excited about doing things to help oneself, and if you're not careful you end up spending your entire life dashing from hospital to homoeo-

*The 1st point on the kidney meridian is situated on the ball of the foot and can sometimes be quite painful.

177

path, from osteopath or organic gardener, with just enough time in between to do your relaxation exercises and grate a few carrots. In the early stages of any programme it is natural to spend rather a lot of time on it, but as the weeks, then the months, and finally the years, go by we must take stock of the situation. To begin with you may find yourself fitting your life into the treatments, but the goal is towards fitting the treatments into your life. A good self-help therapy is just a matter of what you can stand. If we don't end up with a life-style that is worth having then something has gone wrong somewhere along the line.

The good news is that once you start looking for ways to heal yourself you will be amazed at the scope and variety of things available to you. You will never be able to do them all and this means that there's always something else to try. Something that was unavailable or unlikely, or too daft or · dangerous last year, may present itself as a sensible possibility at another time.

Does this mean 1986 will be a bad year for toads we ask ourselves?

For further information please contact:
The Bristol Cancer Help Centre,
Grove House,
Cornwallis Grove
Clifton
Bristol BS8 4PG
Tel: 0272 743216

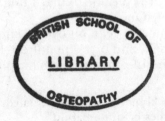